THE DIABETES-FREE COOKBOOK & EXERCISE GUIDE

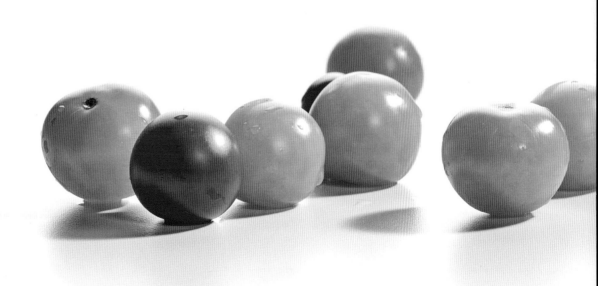

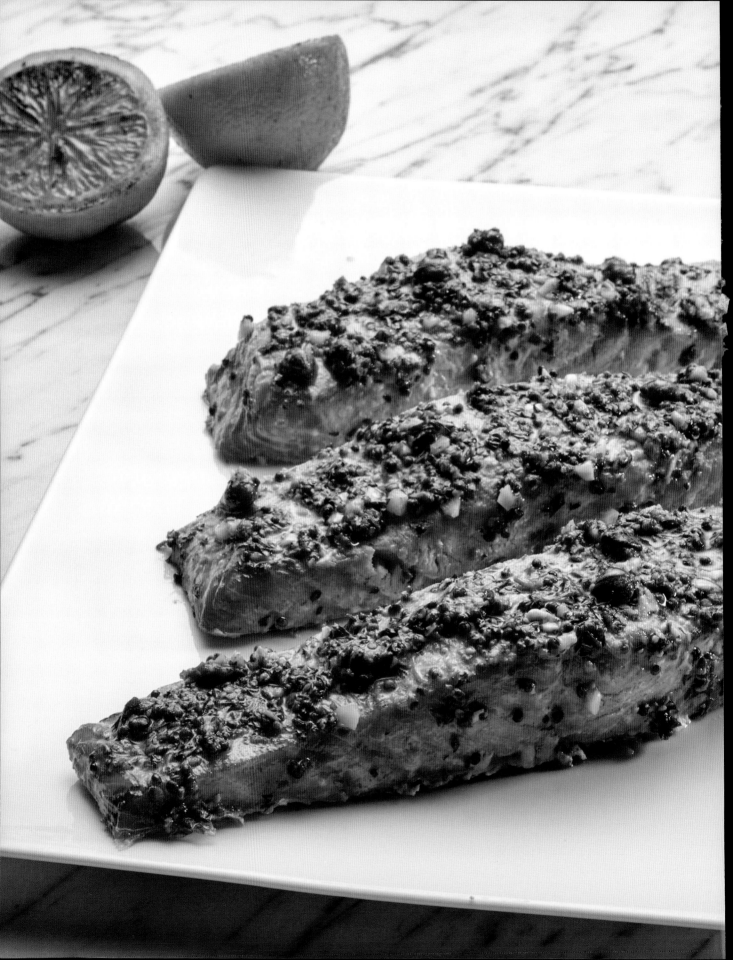

THE
DIABETES-FREE
COOKBOOK & EXERCISE GUIDE

DR. JOHN M. POOTHULLIL, MD, FRCP
WITH CHEF COLLEEN CACKOWSKI

NEW INSIGHTS PRESS

Editorial Direction and Editing: Rick Benzel
Recipes: Chef Colleen Cackowski
Warm Salad Dressings Recipes: Diya Loney
Copyediting: Julie Simpson, OnWords & UpWords!
Creative Director: Susan Shankin
Creative Consultant: Elizabeth Lenthall
Cover Design: Susan Shankin and Elizabeth Lenthall
Interior Book Design: Susan Shankin & Associates
Photography: Anthony Nex
Food Stylist: Diane Elander
Prop Stylist: Kristine Nex

Published by New Insights Press, Los Angeles, CA

Printed in China
Distributed by SCB Distributors

ISBN: 979-8-9860163-4-4 (Hardcover)
ISBN: 979-8-9860163-7-5 (eBook)

Library of Congress Control Number: 2023937479

CONTENTS

INTRODUCTION

There may be several reasons you find yourself interested in this book. Perhaps as someone with Type 2 diabetes who is taking a medication or injecting insulin you are also looking for new ways to control your blood sugar because you found it impossible to avoid foods you love.

Or perhaps you are one of the estimated 96 million people in the United States with prediabetes or a family history of diabetes.

Maybe you are simply looking for a lifestyle change that will benefit your overall wellness through diet and exercise.

Whatever your reasons for wanting to read this book, I can help you in two ways. First, as a retired medical doctor committed to reducing the dangerous health consequences of diabetes in America, I have teamed up with a professional chef who has created fantastic-tasting recipes that will help keep your blood sugar low. Second, I have compiled a variety of very simple and brief exercises that you can do to keep your body in condition.

Diet and exercise are the true keys to preventing or even reversing Type 2 diabetes—and I will explain why. I will also show how anyone can learn to change their eating habits, and why it is so important.

It is difficult for some to stop eating foods they love. They know they should make a change, and they may commit in their mind to eating less at each meal or to giving up foods they know are unhealthy for them. But pure willpower can diminish after a short time, and so most people fall back into their usual eating patterns, willing to live with their high blood sugar or diabetes without thinking about the consequences.

However, I am convinced that you can make a change in your eating habits, and this book can help. What sets this book apart from many others is that we have created a set of meals and desserts that are easy to make and adopt into your routines. They are also super tasty and attractive to your taste buds. Once you try these recipes, you will see that you can indeed eat great meals while at the same time keeping your blood sugar in check. The key is to eat foods that do not cause your blood sugar to spike so high that it takes hours to return to the normal blood sugar range. That is how you begin moving away from being prediabetic or fully diabetic. With meals like these, you can even begin to lower your blood sugar enough to reverse your diagnosed Type 2 diabetes.

How I Became Interested in Diabetes & What I Found Out

I am a retired medical doctor, having practiced for 35 years. I didn't practice endocrinology—the medical specialty that deals with diabetes. But that allowed me to study diabetes from a different perspective and champion a different methodology for people to avoid or reverse it.

While I was in medical school, endocrinology professors told us to believe, as they did themselves, that Type 2 diabetes is a hormonal disease caused by "insulin resistance." I had no reason to dispute this.

Towards the end of my training, I became aware of one of my relatives who was diagnosed with Type 2 diabetes. She was taking insulin to control her blood sugar. Her husband, a professor in a medical school, adjusted her insulin dosage to keep her blood sugar level within an acceptable range. Nevertheless, a few years later, she had to have one of her legs amputated due to reduced blood supply to her leg—a well-known complication of Type 2 diabetes in many adults. I thought her doctor would change her diabetes medication because taking insulin had not stopped her leg complication. To my surprise though, her doctor continued the same line of treatment using insulin. Within a few more months, she had to have the other leg amputated.

I started paying more attention to people who were on insulin to treat their Type 2 diabetes. To my shock, I found others who suffered severe consequences. One friend who was a trained scientist had to have three toes amputated, one after another, after keeping his blood sugar level within normal limits for years using insulin. I soon learned about similar experiences among many acquaintances who lost their vision and others who lost kidney function.

I wondered how this could be. Despite taking medications or injecting insulin, I saw that diabetic patients still suffered the consequences of long-term diabetes. About 25 years ago, I began intently studying the medical literature on hunger, weight gain, obesity, and diabetes.

Through my research, I came to a surprising conclusion—*the theory of "insulin resistance" was illogical and remained scientifically unproven.* I knew I was going against tradition. This theory, however, is what endocrinologists believe in and is the rationale they use to keep prescribing medications and insulin injections to diabetic patients.

So what might cause high blood sugar and diabetes?

I soon came to realize that the answer is staring us right in the face. It is our ***modern diet,*** heavily filled with complex carbohydrates that flood the bloodstream with glucose (sugar). Among so many cultures around the world, the modern diet is the only common denominator that can possibly explain the global increase in the incidence of high blood sugar and Type 2 diabetes. I do not believe that more and more humans are evolving to be insulin resistant. The body produces over 50 hormones, so why would it become resistant to just one? I also know that no genetic defect has ever been discovered that links to Type 2 diabetes.

I suggest that the rising incidence of diabetes began after the "Green Revolution" of the 1960s. New technologies and fertilizers increased the farming of cultivated grains, and governments around the world began subsidizing grain production to ensure enough food for their populations. New milling technologies and lower shipping costs made grain-flour products cheap and easily available. Americans especially, but also people in most Western nations, began consuming a variety of breads, rolls, cakes and pies, doughnuts, pasta, rice, corn, pizza, tortillas . . . and the list goes on.

Why Do Grains and Grain-flour Products Cause Diabetes?

Let me explain why I suggest that our modern diet high in grains and grain-flour products is the most likely trigger for the development of prediabetes or Type 2 diabetes. It is because the typical diet that includes more than 50% of one's daily caloric intake in the form of complex carbohydrates produces a voluminous amount of glucose that the body's cells cannot use on an immediate basis. Some glucose is stored in the liver, then released between meals for the body's energy needs until the next meal.

But here is the key—any unused glucose is transformed into fatty acids that are then stored in one's fat cells. The problem is, each individual has only a certain capacity for fat storage, based on their body type and genetic inheritance. At some point, one's fat cells can literally become full, leaving nowhere for the fatty acids produced from the unused glucose after each meal to be stored.

The result is that the fatty acids remain circulating in the bloodstream. What diabetes specialists seldom admit, however, is that our muscle cells—the largest energy producers in the body—are like a hybrid car. They can burn either glucose or fatty acids for producing energy. Fatty acids can enter right into muscle cells faster and more easily than glucose—and they do, leaving glucose in the bloodstream, thus high blood sugar.

This is what I call the *fatty acid burn switch*. A long-term diet high in complex carbohydrates is what eventually causes chronic high blood sugar—and that eventually becomes Type 2 diabetes.

A diet high in grains and grain-flour products that produce excessive amounts of fatty acids that fill your fat cells is also what leads to weight gain and, for an increasing number of people, obesity. This explains why the majority of people with Type 2 diabetes are overweight or obese as they enter their 40s, 50s, and 60s. But this same diet also explains why we are seeing children as young as 12 and teens become overweight, obese, and even diabetic.

Nevertheless, diabetes can also occur in thin people, simply because they have a small number of fat cells, which leaves them no room to store excess fatty acids. They too can undergo the fatty acid burn switch, creating high blood sugar and diabetes. In many developing countries, such as India, an increasing number of people with Type 2 diabetes are not considered to be extremely overweight. In addition, in Western countries 15% of people with Type 2 diabetes are not considered overweight.

The same biological mechanism of the fatty acid burn switch also explains why a pregnant woman with no previous history of diabetes can develop gestational diabetes. Simply put, when a pregnant woman fills up her fat storage capacity, her muscles switch to burning fatty acids, leaving glucose in the bloodstream. This explanation is in contrast to the present situation, in which endocrinologists have absolutely no hypothesis to explain the development of "insulin resistance" in lean or pregnant diabetics.

Support for Why Diet – Not Medication – Is the Key to Moderating Diabetes

Here is something odd that supports what I am telling you about the *real* cause of high blood sugar and diabetes. You will usually hear that today's medical advice recommends that people with diabetes eat a low carbohydrate diet.

This advice comes from mainstream endocrinologists who support the insulin resistance theory. Although on one hand they recognize that a low-carb diet plays some role in controlling high blood sugar, though they don't know why, on the other hand they tell their patients to continue taking diabetes medications or injecting insulin.

In my view, these doctors are still largely counting on medications as the answer to controlling blood sugar; and they are doing so only because the insulin resistance theory is what they learned in medical school. They are unable to admit this theory is wrong, yet they accept a clear connection between a low carbohydrate diet and low blood sugar.

I am not suggesting that you cannot achieve a low blood sugar level using medications. You can, at least for a while. But what I am saying is that the medication/insulin injection approach has two serious flaws.

First, it is difficult to maintain a desired blood glucose level using medications such as insulin. Your blood sugar level is actually a moving target. Throughout the day, and especially after each meal, it changes depending on what you ate. It swings upwards for about two hours after you eat a meal, then slowly descends. This forces someone with high blood sugar to keep measuring the level of their blood glucose. This is why diabetics who inject insulin must decide how much insulin to inject before and after each meal, or even throughout the day.

The second flaw is what I told you about above. There is absolutely no doubt any longer that, despite taking diabetes medications or injecting insulin, a large percentage of diabetics still end up with one or more of the serious consequences of diabetes: loss of kidney function (which leads to permanent dialysis), loss of vision, and/or nerve damage to limbs (which results in amputation of toes or legs). Yet endocrinologists still prefer to treat diabetes using medications or insulin injections instead of dietary changes. This is tragic.

For these reasons, I suggest to you that it is far better to control your blood sugar level by regulating what you eat. Let me put it this way: if you don't put glucose (carbohydrates) into your mouth, you won't need to worry about having high blood sugar. Doesn't this make logical sense to you? The fact is that cultivated grains or foods made with them are not necessary for healthy living.

 You may not completely understand the science behind what I have just explained. But that is okay. If you want to learn more about that science, click on the QR code to see an animation video titled "Challenging Your Assumptions about Type 2 Diabetes" that illustrates the concept of the fatty acid burn switch. You can also read more about "authentic weight," weight gain, and obesity in the Appendix section of this book where I answer a number of FAQs.

Proof that Dietary Changes Can Help

As I was writing this book, an observational study was published in the British Medical Journal *Nutrition* that showed that 77% of a doctor's patients who followed a lower-carbohydrate diet without medications experienced remission of Type 2 diabetes within one year. However, over the next fifteen years some reverted back to their old ways of eating and the overall remission rate dropped to 51%. These results are impressive and meaningful.

The remission of Type 2 diabetes with a drug-free dietary change cited in this study supports my suggestion that "overnutrition" (eating too much carbohydrate), rather than insulin resistance, is responsible for the elevation of blood sugar leading to the development of Type 2 diabetes. The key to lowering blood sugar level without the use of medications is to reduce the intake of food products which upon digestion release glucose into the blood stream. In our modern day meals, the main culprit is complex carbohydrates primarily coming from grains and grain-flour products.

Try These Recipes for Just One Month

For now, what counts most is recognizing that *your diet is the single most important factor you can control to lower your blood sugar*—and even potentially to prevent or reverse Type 2 diabetes. If you are willing to try altering your diet for just a few weeks, you will see your blood sugar level go down, you may lose a few pounds, and you will feel healthier and more active.

I have already written two books about diabetes in which I explain why I believe the insulin resistance theory is incorrect and why the modern diet high in complex carbohydrates is most certainly the cause of high blood sugar and diabetes. In those books, I provided general information about how to eat for nutrition—cutting out carbs and emphasizing fresh, seasonal vegetables, fruits, and nuts, plus, if desired, a variety of meats, fish, and dairy products. But my readers kept asking me to tell them more precisely what they should eat and how they should cook.

I therefore concluded that it was time to do a cookbook with great recipes to keep your blood sugar level down. Here you will find breakfast, lunch, dinner, snack, and dessert recipes **with minimal use of grains or grain flours.** My objective is not to avoid grains completely but to substantially lower the amount of complex carbohydrate consumed in your diet. These recipes were created by a wonderfully creative nutritionist and chef, Colleen Cackowski, who put her heart and soul into crafting mouth-watering, flavorful meals that are easy and fun to make. You will be amazed at how various ingredients like black beans or riced cauliflower can be mixed with other ingredients to create the flavors and mouth-textures you enjoy.

For the most part, these recipes do not require many special ingredients; most of what you will need you can find at a typical chain grocery store, such as Walmart, Kroger, Albertsons, Trader Joe's, Food Lion, Giant, Publix, Meijer, Whole Foods, or from Amazon.

The greatest advantage of these recipes is that you will not lose your enjoyment of eating or be told to follow a lot of restrictions. For example, these recipes do not show how many calories are in them. My belief is that most people have enough fat stored up in the body to have the energy they need to make it through any given day. Counting calories makes little sense for the average person—and most people struggle to stay within a calorie count anyway. What is more important is that we eat to acquire the nutrients the cells of the body need and that we learn to become more conscious of our eating behaviors.

Although the recipes show how many servings they make, neither Chef Colleen nor I know how much nutrient your body needs when you sit down to eat. Your brain, on the other hand, knows what your body needs and will create the sensation of enjoyment when you consume a food that contains the needed nutrients. More importantly, your brain reduces the intensity of enjoying that food when a sufficient amount has been eaten. In my view, the most effective guideline is thus to eat whatever you enjoy but also pay attention to that arc of enjoyment and loss of enjoyment. To do this, you need to chew your food thoroughly; this is necessary to release the nutrients in your mouth at a rate at which your taste buds and olfactory sensors can record and report their findings to the control centers in the brain. If you pay attention to this "enjoyment / less enjoyment" cycle, you don't need to pre-measure how much you eat.

I invite you to use this book as a stepping stone to a new lifestyle of healthy eating. Begin by using the recipes for just one month as a starting point. Each recipe in this cookbook is composed of ingredients that will not cause your blood sugar to elevate too high or for too long after eating. In this way, you can achieve a more stable blood sugar level throughout the day. You're bound to notice a difference in just a few weeks.

What is most important is for you to believe that you can control your blood sugar and your destiny starting right now. If you are feeling anxious about making all your meals using these recipes, do not worry. Keep the book in your kitchen as a gentle reminder and aim to use some of the recipes to make at least half your meals over the next 30 days. While perhaps not as effective as a complete overhaul of your diet would be, it will be a good start in your effort to lower your blood sugar through your diet. If you can achieve at least a modest level of blood sugar reduction in the coming 30 days, you may be encouraged to cook entirely using these recipes in the following days.

I know it is not easy for many people to give up foods they enjoy, especially those "comfort foods" they have been eating since childhood. But in general, these recipes do not ask you to forego much, other than avoiding carbohydrate-heavy meals. The main suggestion I hope you will follow is to avoid eating the same amount of certain key items—breads, tortillas, pizza, rice, corn, and grain-flour sweets and desserts—as you may have eaten before. I assure you: you won't starve making these recipes, because we have included meals and desserts that will give you the same feeling of satisfaction you are used to. Perhaps even more.

Of course, you may make some missteps or experience anxiety about changing your food preferences. You may find yourself slipping and backsliding multiple times, returning to consuming fast foods, pizza, pastries, donuts, and muffins. You may just cave in and give up on trying these recipes, accepting that your life is easier if you just keep taking your medication to control your blood sugar. You may find it hard to ignore that your past attempts of dietary changes did not help you to accomplish your goal.

Your feeling this way is understandable because a fundamental change in your dietary practices is often painful and challenging to sustain. You may have come to believe that because of your family history—other family members who have diabetes—that you too are not likely to escape diabetes for the rest of your life.

However, keep in mind that science has not found any genetic cause for Type 2 diabetes. Meanwhile, my hypothesis is supported by scientific, logical evidence, that the modern carbohydrate-heavy diet is what triggers high blood sugar and Type 2 diabetes.

At moments when you are feeling hesitant and apprehensive about making the dietary changes I suggest, remember that the best guarantee of preserving the functions of your kidneys, keeping your eyesight, and avoiding amputation of your limbs is by controlling your blood sugar through lifestyle changes—particularly your diet—rather than by resorting to a lifetime of medications such as insulin. I assure you that as you take control of what you can accomplish on your own, many of the fears of a recurrence of demoralizing dietary failures of the past will vanish and you will feel emboldened.

Add 12 Simple Exercises to Create a New Lifestyle

A complementary component to the recipes in this book is a set of twelve simple exercises you can do in the comfort of your own home or anywhere. I chose to include these because people with Type 2 diabetes are often adults who do not exercise enough relative to their age. Let's face it: as we age, we're no longer "spring chickens," full of the energy to exercise an hour or more each day. In fact, the older we get, the harder it is to burn calories as we did when we were younger. Most older adults lose muscle mass (notice, for instance, how your leg muscles are thinner). This means that a half hour of exercise for a man or woman older than 40 burns far fewer calories than for a man or woman younger than 40.

To go along with the printed exercise instructions in this book, I also produced a series of animated videos that show you how to do these twelve movements. While you may prefer to do physical activity outdoors—such as walking, running, cycling, or swimming—those can be challenging for a lot of people, especially if you are busy, or the weather conditions don't allow it, or if you are confined to your home for any reason. I propose this set of twelve easy-to-do exercises that you can do inside your own home at any time. Some examples:

If you find you are bored or when you are just sitting around on the couch, you can do the deep breathing exercise, paying attention to the movement of air through your nose and the movement of your chest wall muscles. It's a great exercise to do when you are watching TV as well, especially to pass the time during commercials.

Toe taps are an excellent activity when you are a passenger in a car, train, or airplane, or when there is a dull moment while you are sitting and watching a stage or sporting event, during a meeting, or while waiting for an appointment. You could also do toe taps in the standing position when you are forced to stand in a train or subway car, or any slow-moving commuter vehicle, using one leg after another.

You can do the leg-related exercises every morning before you get out of your bed. In fact, every time you lie down, you have an opportunity to do one or more of the leg exercises. If you have a history of feeling dizzy when you stand up suddenly after being on your back for some time, this could be due to a condition called postural hypotension. Doing leg exercises before getting up to a sitting position or doing toe tapping in the sitting position before standing up, could speed delivery of blood to your brain and limit the degree of dizziness from postural hypotension.

Over time, you may find other opportunities to put these exercises into practice.

Organization of the Book

Part 1 of this book includes a brief introduction from Chef Colleen Cackowski, followed by the recipes. Each recipe includes the list of ingredients in the order in which you use them when cooking, followed by the specific cooking instructions. Many recipes also suggest variations on a theme, inviting you to alter the recipe with slightly different ingredients for a change-up now and then.

Part 2 provides written explanations for how to do the exercises. There is a QR code that you can capture with your phone's camera; it will take you right to a page on the internet where you can watch the animated video showing you how to perform each exercise.

Part 3 offers a five-step program that I created to help you learn to stay motivated to control your blood sugar and your weight.

In the Appendix to this book, I have included a wealth of additional information adapted from my two prior books about diabetes: *Eat, Chew, Live: 4 Revolutionary Ideas to Prevent Diabetes, Lose Weight and Enjoy Food* and *Diabetes: The Real Cause and the Right Cure, 8 Steps to Reverse Type 2 Diabetes.*

PART 1

80 Delicious Recipes to Support Blood Sugar Control

BY CHEF COLLEEN CACKOWSKI

As Dr. John discussed in the introduction, Type 2 diabetes needs to be recognized as a "life-style" disease—meaning that your conscious choices affect how you maintain your state of health. Your lifestyle choices include your physical activity, the amount you sleep, how you deal with stress, and most importantly, the food you eat.

In this book, you will find recipes I have created that focus on foods known to stabilize blood sugar levels. When you eat a lot of carbohydrates (such as bread, rice, pasta, pizza, tortillas, baked goods, etc.) and processed foods, you can easily see that your blood sugar levels will spike. That's why in these recipes I share fiber-rich, natural foods and lean proteins that will help keep your blood sugar at a more even level and prevent dramatic swings. I emphasize "low glycemic index" ingredients, by which I mean foods that are rated on the glycemic index to raise your blood sugar the most slowly.

There are other benefits of eating a diet high in foods close to nature, by which I mean vegetables, beans, legumes, nuts, and seeds. Your intestinal bacteria colony will be more in balance and you will feel less lethargic after eating.

We all make choices. Over time, these choices become habits, which can bring us either further away from our health goals or closer to them. My secret to maintaining a long-term, healthy relationship with food lies in making healthy and nutritious meals that taste delicious. It may take you a little time at first, but the investment in your health is worth the extra effort.

I created these recipes to be free of the most common perpetrators of a sickly lifestyle: wheat, sugar, corn, rice, and other high-glycemic carbohydrates, such as white potatoes. Will you feel deprived if you make these recipes a regular part of your meals? Absolutely not! These recipes are brimming with flavor and chock full of nutrition. As you sample these foods, meal after meal, your body will start to recognize and value true nourishment. You may be surprised to notice that you no longer have the same taste for empty calories that you used to crave.

The Glycemic Index

This index was created in 1981 by Professor David Jenkins at the University of Toronto to identify how fast a food item raises blood glucose levels. It works on a scale of 0 to 100, with pure glucose being 100. The score of each particular food is determined by how much and what type of carbohydrate it contains, as well as by how quickly that carbohydrate is released into the body and whether the food is cooked or raw. As individuals may differ in how fast their body absorbs glucose, the index is an approximation of the average rate.

Balancing the Five Flavors

In Dr. John's book *Eat, Chew, Live: 4 Revolutionary Ideas to Prevent Diabetes, Lose Weight and Enjoy Food*, he discusses how the taste buds in the mouth and smell sensors in the nasal cavity relay the sensations of taste and flavor to your brain, which can then track the nutrients you ingest. In professional cuisine, we also pay attention to the notion that the mouth can distinguish five flavors, which is how you interpret your enjoyment of food.

Flavor	Food Examples
Sweet	Sweet potatoes, avocados, squashes, carrots, onions, parsnips, cashews, chestnuts, honey, and most fruits
Sour	Lemons, limes, kiwi, pickles, vinegar, and sauerkraut, as well as cultured dairy products like buttermilk and sour cream
Salty	Celery, seaweeds, miso, eggs, seafood, prosciutto, feta, tamari, and brined vegetables such as olives and pickles
Spicy/ Pungent	Onions, scallions, ginger, garlic, peppers, chilies, radishes, wasabi, mushrooms, and many spices
Bitter	Many dark leafy greens like kale, dandelion, mustard, collards, and arugula, as well as bitter melon, coffee, dark chocolate, tea, and parsley

Although I am known for my recipes and work in the raw food industry, I am not advocating a completely raw food diet. Most of the recipes I present here are cooked. However, one of my most important cooking lessons came from one of my mentors, Cherie Soria, "The Mother of Gourmet Raw Food." She created some of the most delicious and healthy dishes in the world of raw food. She taught me the importance of balancing the five flavors. Not every dish will contain all five flavors, but any time you can include as many of them as possible— in a delicious balance—you will create a tasty dish that has wide appeal.

Use the recipes in this book as your starting point to experiment with the five flavors. I always advocate that, as you are cooking, you should taste your food to gauge if it includes all five flavors—or as many of them as makes sense. If you need to adjust the balance, think of a food that contains the missing flavor. Decide if it would work to add that ingredient into the mix. For example, you could top your non-bitter food with a small sprig of parsley to incorporate a bitter flavor. It may take some practice, but ultimately, it will be worth the effort!

Cooking with Herbs and Spices

The human attraction to herbs and spices may not be simply that they add to the taste of our food. In fact, we may enjoy the taste of herbs and spices because they supply us with micronutrients needed by the body. One can obtain many micronutrients from different herbs and spices. For example, antioxidants in spices such as saffron, turmeric, and oregano can counter some of the negative health effects of additives and preservatives that you may not be able to avoid completely.

Keep in mind that the beneficial concentration of each nutrient contained in a particular herb or spice is unknown. There is no standardization of herbs and spices, in general. Also, the concentration of individual nutrients could vary with the location of production, cultivation style, weather and water availability, and processing methods. The fact is that, at present, we have no test to identify the quantity of each nutrient the body is lacking when a person sits down to eat. Even if that were possible, one does not know how much of each element/nutrient is present in the food item.

Spices are underused in most American kitchens. People who live in the Middle East, India, China, and Japan usually cook with a wide variety of herbs and spices, as they do much more than add flavor to a dish. Yet another benefit of using spices is it helps you reduce the quantity of salt, which today is being consumed in much higher quantities than recommended for human beings.

Note that spices are mostly fat soluble, which means they dissolve better in fat or oil. When food is agitated and warmed in the mouth during chewing, those volatile fat molecules move into the nasal cavity to stimulate your smell receptors. This allows you to appreciate the full flavor of the meal, similar to appreciating the fragrance of a perfume sprayed in the air. Some spices also contain compounds that can have a beneficial effect on mood, cognition, digestion, and more. For example:

- **Spicy pepper.** It aids digestion, stimulates blood circulation, and has antibacterial properties.

- **Cinnamon.** It may be able to help lower blood sugar and support healthy cholesterol levels. There are two kinds: cassia and Ceylon cinnamon. Cassia contains more coumarin which has been shown to damage the liver in high doses, so check your labels and choose Ceylon cinnamon for regular use. Saigon or Vietnamese cinnamon has a stronger flavor and aroma than other varieties so I do like to use it for special treats, but it is a species of cassia cinnamon, so usage should not exceed 1 teaspoon per day. Cinnamon can influence brain function by boosting concentration and attention.

- **Ginger.** It can help with gastrointestinal distress, contains anti-inflammatory and analgesic agents, and adds amazing olfactory and taste benefits.

- **Turmeric.** Curcumin, the active ingredient in turmeric, has anti-inflammatory and antioxidant benefits. These benefits can be particularly helpful in delaying aging and fighting some chronic diseases as well as being good for your brain. It also stimulates the release of serotonin, a natural mood enhancer.

Feel free to use herbs like these with any dish. Instead of adding extra salt and butter, use spices to bring out the best in your foods!

The Role of Sweetness in the Body

The mistake we often make when we crave sweetness (often accompanied by a need for instant gratification) is that we end up consuming too much processed sugar or other complex carbohydrates to fulfill that longing. But did you know there are so many other options to satisfy your sweet tooth? Through these recipes, I will teach you to use healthy food-based sweeteners to satisfy your body's cravings for sweet flavor.

Sweet flavors make up most of our normal meals. Think about it . . . Breakfast in the Western world is typically cereal, a muffin, a donut, a croissant, sugar-laden yogurt, or some other carb-based food product like pancakes, waffles, or toast. Lunch is often a sandwich, pizza (bread), or maybe a hot dog or hamburger (wrapped in bread) or some noodles. And then for dinner, we want rice, potato, or pasta to go with our protein and a small portion of vegetables. And this is also often accompanied by bread or rolls.

All of these complex carb-based food items qualify as "sweet" in the flavor index because on digestion they yield glucose. The problem is, the quantity is way out of balance for good health, and the quality is usually lacking. The fact is, for thousands of years, humans used to eat simpler, less processed foods. The majority of foods now available in a standard supermarket had not been invented until maybe 100 years ago or less. In choosing these boxed and packaged convenience foods, we have created a huge health crisis. We need to get back to eating more natural ingredients that our bodies know how to digest and assimilate to return to an optimal state of health.

It can be life-changing to learn to use natural flavors in foods to shape your health. As you become healthier, your body will reflect the changes with respect to your tastes and cravings. You may be surprised to wake up one morning and have absolutely no desire for that tray of pastries someone brought to the office!

To get started on this journey, take a moment to step back and observe your habits. When you crave sweetness, try what nature has provided to us in their "natural packaging," i.e., the sweetness of fruits. In doing this, you will experience reduced sugar cravings as a wonderful and beneficial side effect! Moreover, eating three different varieties of fruits a day can help the body acquire many nutrients to boost your immune system.

Getting the Most from Your Food

Whether you have prediabetes, diabetes, or you want to lower your risk of developing diabetes, here is a list of foods that you can begin incorporating into a regular part of a nutritious diet to help you lower your blood sugar. I have shaped many of the recipes in this book around these great foods because they help maintain healthy blood sugar levels. The explanations of these foods below will also clarify many questions people often have about certain food ingredients and why I particularly recommend some items over others.

Apple cider vinegar. For recipes that require vinegar, apple cider vinegar is usually my vinegar of choice due to the health benefits it offers. For hundreds of years, using naturally fermented apple cider vinegar medicinally as well as for culinary purposes has been successful. Even Hippocrates, the father of modern medicine, used vinegar as a tonic for energy and as a healing elixir. Apple cider vinegar is a completely natural product, resulting from a series of fermentation processes of the fruit's juices. In order to maximize the benefits, look for apple cider vinegar that has not been pasteurized, filtered, refined, or distilled. It should be made from cold pressed, organically grown whole apples, to which no chemicals or preservatives have been added. Good quality vinegar should have a slightly cloudy appearance from the naturally occurring strands of enzymes and proteins.

Animal proteins (meat, chicken, fish). Animal proteins do not have a significant impact on blood sugar. Many people with diabetes include them as part of their healthy diet. This is fine so long as you are mindful of the quantity and quality of the proteins you choose. For optimal health, most of your plate should consist of plant-based foods—as close to nature as possible (not processed). You will get the most nutrition and health benefits this way. Adding a small serving of animal protein will additionally support balanced blood sugar levels for some people.

Note that eating too much animal protein forces the liver to convert some of the amino acids into glucose, defeating the goal of lowering your blood sugar. You may have to experiment to find out how much protein is right for you and if you really need so much animal protein; you may find your body can live with more plant-based protein or wants a combination of the two. When you choose to have animal protein, opt for grass-fed, free-range, or organic meats and wild-caught fish as much as possible.

Arrowroot. It's a starchy vegetable commonly used as a thickener in desserts and baked goods. It is easily digestible and provides calcium, magnesium, and some fiber. Arrowroot may benefit people who choose a gluten-free diet and those managing blood sugar and weight. Arrowroot is a healthier alternative to ingredients like cornstarch, tapioca, or potato starch, which can be high glycemic. Arrowroot powder and arrowroot flour are the same thing. It can also be called arrowroot starch.

Artichokes. They are full of healthy soluble and prebiotic fibers, supporting healthy digestion and helping to lower post-meal glucose levels.

Avocados. As a fruit that is low in carbohydrates, avocados have little effect on blood sugar levels. They also contain a lot of fiber. The combination of low sugar and high fiber, along with healthy fats, make avocados an ideal food for people who want to balance blood sugar.

Beans. Also called pulses, beans are full of fiber, which slows digestion and blood sugar spikes. Beans contain plant-based protein, so between the protein and fiber, eating about a half cup serving of beans will help slow down how quickly your blood sugar rises. Because they also contain vitamins and minerals, they can be a good choice for people looking to control their Type 2 diabetes.

Broth. You can make soup recipes by simply using good quality water and herb seasonings to create your own broth, but I also recommend starting with a quality pre-made broth for added nutrients and flavor. Whether you use beef, chicken, or vegetable broth, it can add a beautiful savory component to your dish. When selecting a broth, I usually look for something free range or organic, with reduced sodium.

Cacao. You may be confused about the difference between cacao powder and cocoa powder. Both these products come from the *Theobroma cacao* tree. This tree produces large, pod-like fruits, each containing 20–60 beans, which are the starting point for anything "chocolate." While the use of the names is not consistent, typically "cacao" powder is reserved for the raw chocolate powder that is extracted from cacao beans after the beans have dried and been fermented. "Cocoa" powder is used for the powder that is extracted after the beans have been roasted. Generally, raw cacao powder is less processed, will contain more antioxidants and nutrition (magnesium, selenium, chromium, manganese) and contains no additives. Cocoa powder, which is generally used for baking, often contains other chemical additives. I use raw cacao powder in my recipes. Cocoa powder can be substituted but be aware that it has a different flavor profile so other elements of the recipe may need to be adjusted to compensate for the difference in flavor (bitterness).

Cauliflower. It contains a small amount of natural sugar. Cauliflower is low on the glycemic index and high in fiber. It also contains vitamins B6 and C, and magnesium. It can be a great replacement for rice or mashed potatoes. Cauliflower can help promote healthy digestion while encouraging the growth of healthy bacteria. Like everything else, make sure to include cauliflower in your diet in moderation to avoid digestive distress.

Chickpeas. Also called garbanzo beans, they are well-known for having a low glycemic index, making them a good choice for diabetics. They are an excellent source of non-animal protein, which is also suitable for vegans and vegetarians. And they are brimming with vitamins and minerals. Chickpeas are naturally gluten-free and versatile. You can put them in salads, use them as a side dish, add them to soups, or use their flour to make healthier versions of bread and pasta.

Chickpea flour is a gluten-free flour that is gaining popularity as an alternative to wheat flour. Chickpea flour is neutral tasting and can be used as a binding agent, as a thickener, or to combine with other ingredients for making gluten-free breads.

Coconut. This is a dairy-free, gluten-free, and paleo- and keto-friendly ingredient used in a variety of recipes for its health benefits, as well as its flavor and texture. I often use coconut cream instead of dairy cream in recipes. It has a wonderful, thick, creamy texture and adds a delicious mild flavor as well. I use all forms of coconut throughout this book: coconut oil, coconut milk (a substitute for dairy milk), coconut cream (substitute for dairy cream), coconut butter (the meat of the coconut blended together with the oil), coconut flour, coconut water, coconut aminos (a substitute for soy sauce), coconut sugar, and coconut nectar.

Dates. They are a great way to sweeten foods naturally because they contain a lot of fiber, antioxidants, and minerals to offset their carbs. They do contain sugar so you should enjoy dates sparingly or in moderation, but I love a date stuffed with some almond butter to satisfy a sweet craving every now and then. Medjool dates are the easiest and best variety for the recipes presented here because they are typically large, soft, and easy to blend, but use what you can easily find and what works best for you.

Fiber-rich foods. Fiber is absolutely essential for a healthy body. Dietary fiber is found mainly in fruits, vegetables, legumes (beans), seeds, and nuts. Insoluble fiber is the part of food that enzymes in the human small intestine can't break down, so it passes into the large intestine, where it promotes the growth of healthy bacteria. A healthy bacterial colony in the intestine provides many useful functions, such as preventing intestinal infections, modification of ingested drugs, promoting a healthy immune system, releasing signaling molecules that affect brain function, providing nourishment for intestinal lining cells, and producing gas that is necessary for regular elimination. In fact, absence of fiber intake is a contributing factor in the development of constipation experienced by many who practice intermittent fasting. Fiber is particularly important to diabetics because it helps keep blood sugar levels stable. Many high fiber ingredients are presented here as healthy options, including chia seeds, psyllium husks, and lots of vegetables.

Garlic. It has been shown to reduce blood sugar levels and increase insulin levels in the body. It is one of the rare foods with *no* glycemic index.

Leafy green vegetables. Spinach, kale, cabbage, lettuce, broccoli, and other leafy green vegetables (and green vegetables, in general) are nutritious and very low in calories. Vegetables are extremely important to managing diabetes. They are an excellent source of many vitamins and minerals, which are beneficial for health and the immune system. Rich in omega-3 fatty acids, they also help improve insulin secretion and assist in regulating blood sugar levels. Greens are typically loaded with fiber, which can control hunger and promote overall digestive health. They can easily be added to any meal—toss them into soups, salads, or sandwiches, or include them as a side dish or a main meal. It's important to get some in your diet every day! The body needs over 100 different nutrients for healthy functioning. Eating at least three different vegetables a day can help you to accomplish that, as each type of green contains a different variety of nutrients.

Lentils. They are a good source of vegetable protein and contain a lot of nutrition in the form of vitamins and minerals. They do have carbs, but they are slow to digest by the intestinal enzymes and therefore should not be problematic for most people managing their blood sugar. Lentils are among the best legumes you can eat because of their slow digestion.

Miso paste. It's a fermented soybean product that is packed with protein, vitamins, and minerals. It has many benefits, including the probiotics that your body's inner ecosystem will love. The miso paste I recommend for recipes is a fresh product, usually found in the refrigerated section of a grocery or health food store. One container will keep stable for months in the fridge. I love to take a scoop of miso paste and blend with some warm water to make a nourishing broth in one minute or less! Miso paste is sold in a variety of colors from white to dark. Usually the darker the color, the stronger the flavor, so start with something milder if you've never tried it before.

Mushrooms. They are very low in sugar and carbohydrates. Since they are low on the glycemic index, they are considered to have anti-diabetic properties. They are also rich in selenium and certain B vitamins. Mushrooms are known to produce cell-protective antioxidants, and contain antibacterial and antiviral compounds. Some are being investigated for anti-cancer properties.

Nutritional yeast. It usually looks like pale yellow flakes and naturally contains healthy B vitamins, including thiamine, riboflavin, vitamin B6, and folate. It's a great flavoring agent. Sprinkle on anything; it tastes like cheese, without the dairy!

Nuts. They contain essential unsaturated fatty acids, vitamins, and essential amino acids. Many nuts are good sources of vitamin E, vitamin B12, folate, and minerals such as magnesium, phosphorus, potassium, selenium, and copper.

The nuts used in the recipes in this book are raw, which is how I recommend eating all nuts rather than roasted or salted. Consumed in moderation, nuts can be part of a healthy, whole-foods diet for people with diabetes, unless you have allergies to them. Common tree nuts include cashews, almonds, macadamias, Brazil nuts, hazelnuts, and walnuts.. Eating three different nuts a day can provide the body with a variety of useful nutrients. Note: peanuts belong to the legume family, and so are not truly nuts.

Oats. These are a grain used in some of the recipes, but they contain 20% less carbohydrate than rice, wheat, or corn. Rolled oats have been partially cooked and flattened, so they are milder with a softer texture than steel-cut oats. If desired, you can substitute quinoa flakes for oats to have more protein and fewer carbs in these recipes.

Oils. There are many types of oils. I always recommend using coconut or avocado oil for cooking because they have a high smoke point and therefore retain their molecular integrity at higher temperatures. Other healthy oils, like olive oil, can be included in your diet, but beware. If you heat olive oil, its beneficial compounds start to degrade, and potentially health-harming compounds form. Olive oil is best used on salads or as a drizzle on cooked or steamed foods. I also suggest not to use the commercially produced cooking oils commonly found on grocery store shelves (like canola or vegetable oil). If you have tried unrefined coconut oil and don't like the mild coconutty taste, you can buy refined coconut oil; it contains no flavor and is safe to cook at high temperatures..

Onions. They are a good source of vitamin C, potassium, quercetin, antioxidants, and other micronutrients.

Pesto. Fresh pesto is packed with antioxidants and plays an important role in protecting the body from the harmful effects of oxidative damage. It's easy to make a big batch, then freeze it in an ice cube tray. Then anytime you need a little pesto in a recipe or to spruce up some steamed veggies, you can simply pull out a frozen cube or two and you're all set! When you make your own pesto you have full control over the ingredients so you can add (or not add) the salt/dairy/nuts/herbs that you prefer. If you're not in a pesto-making frame of mind, you can usually get fresh pesto in the refrigerated section of your grocery or find some shelf-stable pesto near the pasta aisle.

Note: If making pesto in advance, you can store it in a sealed glass jar in the refrigerator for up to four days. If you are making pesto ice cubes, store them in an airtight container in the freezer for up to three months. Several recipes in this book call for pesto so it's a great item to have on hand when needed.

Quinoa. This is a seed, not a grain, though it is cooked like a grain. Quinoa is naturally gluten-free and is a good source of many important nutrients, including folate, magnesium, zinc, and iron. It's also rich in protein and fiber, allowing it to be included in diabetic-friendly recipes. I use quinoa flour and quinoa flakes in some recipes when I want to increase the protein/fiber content in place of other forms of flour or oatmeal flakes. There are many types of quinoa including red, black, and white. Usually darker foods have a stronger flavor and somewhat more dense nutritional value. White quinoa has a fluffier texture and milder flavor.

Salt. I recommend that you use mineral salt, not common table salt. Good quality mineral salts include: Himalayan pink salt, Celtic sea salt, Fleur de sel, black salt, or red salt. Be sure to choose salt from a clean source. Kosher salt is OK for cooking but contains fewer minerals. Himalayan pink salt is an ideal culinary salt. It's easy to find, easy to use, and stores well.

Salt is mostly sodium chloride in whatever form it is sold. However, common table salt contains various additives and anti-caking agents, including fluoride, magnesium carbonate, calcium carbonate, and aluminum hydroxide to improve its ability to pour out easily. Some table salts may contain additives such as iodine, iron, folic acid, and fluoride that are used to address a variety of health concerns, especially in the developing world.

Sodium is an essential nutrient for human health. However, excessive salt consumption may increase cardiovascular disease risk in people diagnosed with high blood pressure. The World Health Organization recommends that adults consume less than 2,000 mg (milligrams) of sodium, equivalent to 5 grams of salt, per day. Most people overconsume salt relative to this amount.

Seasoning packages. Store-bought seasoning packets may contain additives of unknown quality and unspecific quantity because there is no standardization. I suggest you make your own mix using your own choice of seasonings, depending on the recipe, without any chemicals or added carbs. It's easy and you can multiply the recipe to make a bigger batch and keep it on hand for future recipes.

Sweet potatoes. They contain a fair amount of carbs; however, they also have protein and fiber, which may help reduce how quickly your blood sugar changes after eating them. If you are going to eat carbs, it's important to choose nutrient-dense carbs that contain fiber as well as vitamins and minerals. Because sweet potatoes do contain fiber and other nutrients, such as potassium, and vitamins A and C, they can be included as part of a healthy diet, more so than white potatoes.

Tahini. It's a thick paste made from sesame seeds that is popular in Middle Eastern dishes. It can be used as a dressing, dip, spread, or condiment. It has a slightly bitter taste but has many health benefits and is versatile in cooking.

Tamari. It's a Japanese sauce made from fermented soybeans. It is a wheat-free version of regular soy sauce that is vegan and gluten-free. You can substitute nama shoyu as an alternative to tamari, which is an unpasteurized version of soy sauce. If you prefer to avoid the soy altogether, try coconut aminos, which is a liquid condiment similar to soy sauce but made from the fermented sap of a coconut palm tree with sea salt. Tamari-type flavoring is useful in dishes as a marinade, dipping sauce (for lettuce wraps or nori rolls), in soup stock, salad dressings, or as a general condiment.

Tomatoes. They are low in total carbohydrates and contain important antioxidants such as beta-carotene and lycopene.

Zucchini. It's very low in calories, and provides vitamins, minerals, and antioxidants, which are important for hormonal regulation and blood sugar stability.

Simple Tips & Tricks

I understand the lure of easy, prepared foods; I am as busy as anyone else. But, delicious, good-quality food is also important to me, so I am careful where I make compromises. Here are a few Tips & Tricks I have learned to make both my food and cooking experience easier:

- For most recipes, assemble all the ingredients first in their measured amounts in their own separate bowls or plates. This makes the process of preparing and cooking the meal easier and more enjoyable than scurrying around your kitchen trying to find items and chop them while cooking part of the recipe.

- Save time by pre-mixing seasoning blends and storing them in a sealed, airtight, glass jar. They last longer in glass, and it makes it easy to add ingredients to your dish quickly.

- Be creative and substitute similar ingredients if you need to, based on your diet or what you have in your pantry. For example, if you don't eat pork bacon, use turkey bacon. In recipes that call for ground beef, you could try ground bison, ground turkey, ground chicken—or even chickpeas.

- If you are short on time and looking to prepare a chicken-based dish, you can start with a sliced or diced pre-cooked rotisserie chicken from your local grocery, instead of starting from scratch.

- Roasting vegetables brings out their sweetness. They taste very different from stewed or boiled versions. In most cases, you can roast in advance and have the ingredient already prepared when you begin the recipe.

- Plating is important! You start to eat with your eyes. Since you are taking the time to make healthy and delicious food from scratch, make its appearance on the plate also attractive by adding a pop of color with a garnish such as a lemon wedge or some sprigs of parsley around the dish.

- Cooking can be a great way to involve your kids in healthy eating and the enjoyment of good food. When children learn how to make delicious dishes at a young age, they will have a valuable skill that lasts a lifetime.

For the ingredients in these recipes, I have tried to mainly use everyday foods that are easy to find in any supermarket. But there are some exceptions; some dishes incorporate special ingredients, either because of the health benefit or because of the unique taste profile that ingredient creates. Spices such as za'atar (a blend), and ajwain seed or carom seed are typically available at more ethnic groceries. Lower carb items such as kelp noodles and grain-free/high protein cereal (such as Catalina Crunch) can usually be found at health food stores. You may be surprised to find other ingredients, like nori seaweed and date sugar, in your local supermarket. Sometimes things are available around you but because you never looked for them before, you might not have realized they were always there. In these modern times, however, we can always find things online as well and have them delivered right to our doors!

A Word on Water

Water is an essential nutrient, the basis of fluids in all living organisms, and a requirement to sustain life. According to a National Institute of Health study published in 2023, adults who stay well-hydrated appear to be healthier, develop fewer chronic conditions, and live longer than those who may not get sufficient fluids.

Our bodies are 70% water and that means that good quality water is more important than food for helping our bodies carry out their normal processes. In fact, your blood is 93 percent water and your muscles are about 75 percent water. As a rule, humans can survive weeks without food, but only a matter of days without water.

Although most people can tolerate a 3–4% decrease in total body water, it could impair cognitive performance in some. A 5–8% decrease can cause fatigue and dizziness. Loss of 10% of total body water can cause physical and mental deterioration along with severe thirst. Dehydration can lead to high levels of sodium ions in the blood.

Water needs to be clean and free of toxins and microbes in order to prevent disease. For me, the ideal water is natural spring water, fresh out of the earth from a clean source. Although experts calculate an average daily intake of 6–9 cups for women and 8–12 cups for men, the amount needed each day really depends on multiple changing factors such as ambient temperature, humidity, level of one's physical activity, exposure to a heat source, and the availability and consumption of water or water-containing items.

A Note on Organic Ingredients in the Recipes

I did not indicate the use of "organic" and non-GMO ingredients throughout the recipes, but I do want to mention that I think these items are helpful and important. For some people, adopting an organic lifestyle is simply too expensive or is too much change all at once. I don't want to deter people from trying these recipes and taking a giant step in the direction of better health.

However, whenever you can lower the load of pesticides and toxins that most conventionally produced food contains, you are doing your body a favor. If your budget is tight, make yourself aware of the "Dirty Dozen" foods that you should always try to buy organic because they are the most compromised: spinach, bell peppers, green beans, kale/collard greens, strawberries, nectarines, apples, grapes, cherries, peaches, pears, and blueberries. Likewise, there is an annual list of the "Clean 15," which are conventionally produced foods that have relatively less contamination: sweet corn, mushrooms, avocados, sweet peas (frozen), asparagus, onions, carrots, cabbage, watermelon, honey dew melons, kiwi, pineapple, papaya, mangoes, and sweet potatoes. The Clean 15 are less critically important for you to spend the extra money on to buy organic. Note, however, that these lists change somewhat each year, so you might search the internet to see if there are any changes from time to time. The point is, make sure you are aware of how your food is being produced whenever possible.

Be Open to Changing Your Eating Habits and Your Life

I know some of these recipes may seem like they require many ingredients or take longer to cook than a microwaved waffle. But you will be preparing food that tastes like you are in a fine restaurant. A few more ingredients—and a little more time—makes a delicious difference.

You need to take action to make a change in your health. If you always do what you've always done, you'll always get what you've always gotten, including high blood sugar and diabetes.

Be open to breaking this cycle. Take charge of your life and health: boldly step in a new direction, one meal at a time. I thank you, but more importantly, your body will thank you!

P.S. Also, a note from Dr. John. He reminds you that if you are going to add any sides to the meals in this book, such as bread or rolls, be sure that they do not exceed 200 calories (based on an average of about 500 to 700 calories for lunch and dinner as suggested by nutrition experts). Although the recipes in this book do not count calories, it is just a given that any grain products you add on your own to the meals herein should not add too many calories.

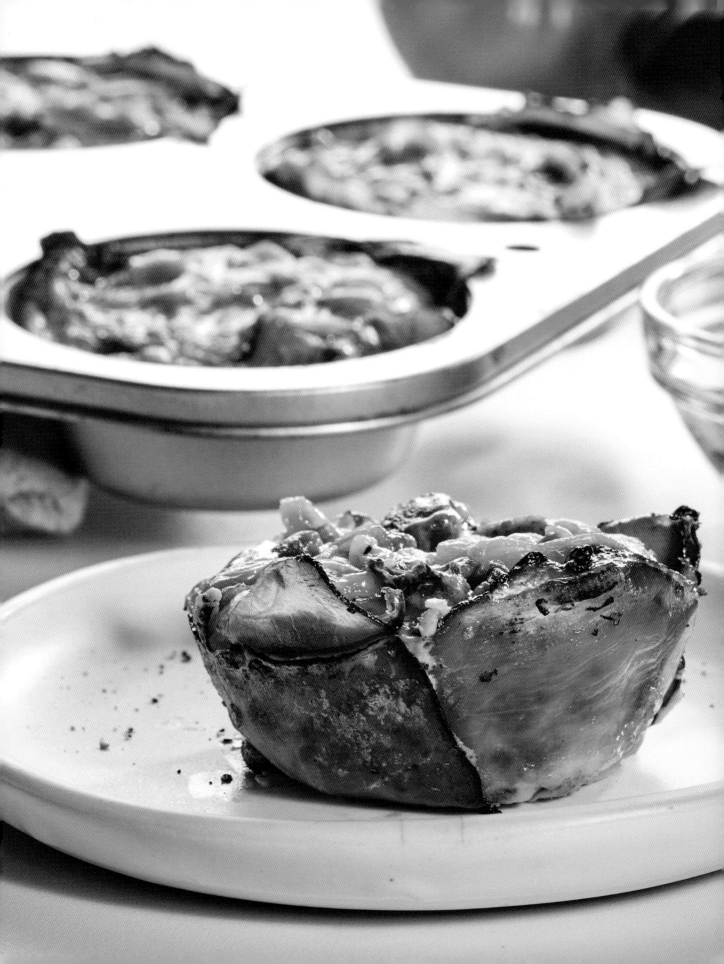

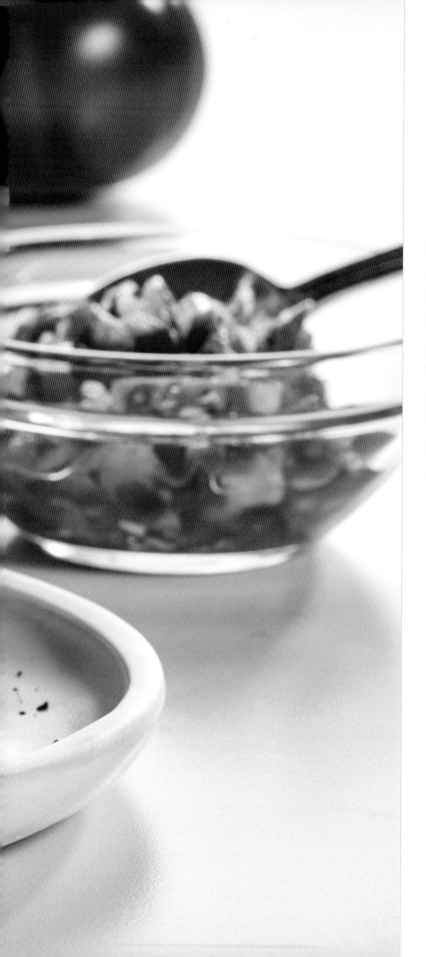

BREAKFASTS

Chewy Breakfast Cookies

Makes 9–10 cookies.

These are great for breakfast or as a post-workout treat. The ultimate grab-and-go item that's easy to make and store for any time hunger strikes!

Ingredients

- 1 large or 2 small bananas, mashed (or ½ cup unsweetened apple sauce or pumpkin puree)
- 1 cup quinoa flakes (or rolled oats)
- ½ cup walnuts, chopped (or your favorite nut)
- ½ cup pumpkin seeds or sunflower seeds
- ½ cup dried fruit-juice sweetened cranberries or raisins
- ½ cup almond butter (or your favorite nut or seed butter)
- 2 Tbsp. chia seeds
- 2-3 Tbsp. real maple syrup (not pancake syrup) or honey
- 2 tsp. cinnamon
- 2 tsp. vanilla
- 1 tsp. ginger powder
- Pinch of salt

Directions

Preheat oven to 350°F. Line a baking tray with parchment paper.

In a bowl, mix all the ingredients together until evenly distributed and your dough sticks together. Start with just 2 Tbsp. of maple syrup or honey. Taste the mixture; add more syrup or honey if you want more sweetness.

Divide your dough into approximately 9–10 portions. Roll each portion of dough into a ball and press down to roughly ½" tall and about 2" across on the baking sheet. Create the cookie shape you want before baking.

Bake for approximately 15–25 minutes, depending on the size of the cookie. They should be light brown when finished and hold together well after they cool.

Notes

- Store in an airtight container for up to a week, or make and freeze.

- You can use rolled oats but I use quinoa flakes to increase the protein and decrease the carbs in this recipe. You can find these online.

Variation

If you don't eat nuts, you can substitute sunflower butter for the nut butter, and seeds instead of chopped nuts.

Beyond this recipe

You can make this as a bar if you'd prefer. Use an 8" x 8" lined baking tin. Bake for the same amount of time as the cookies. Cut into bars after it cools.

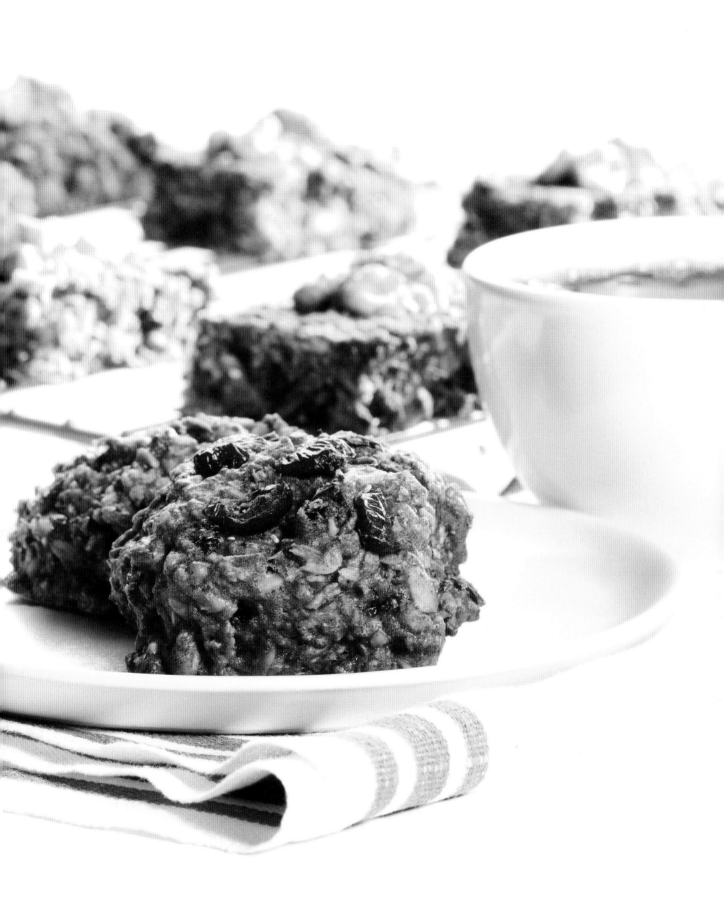

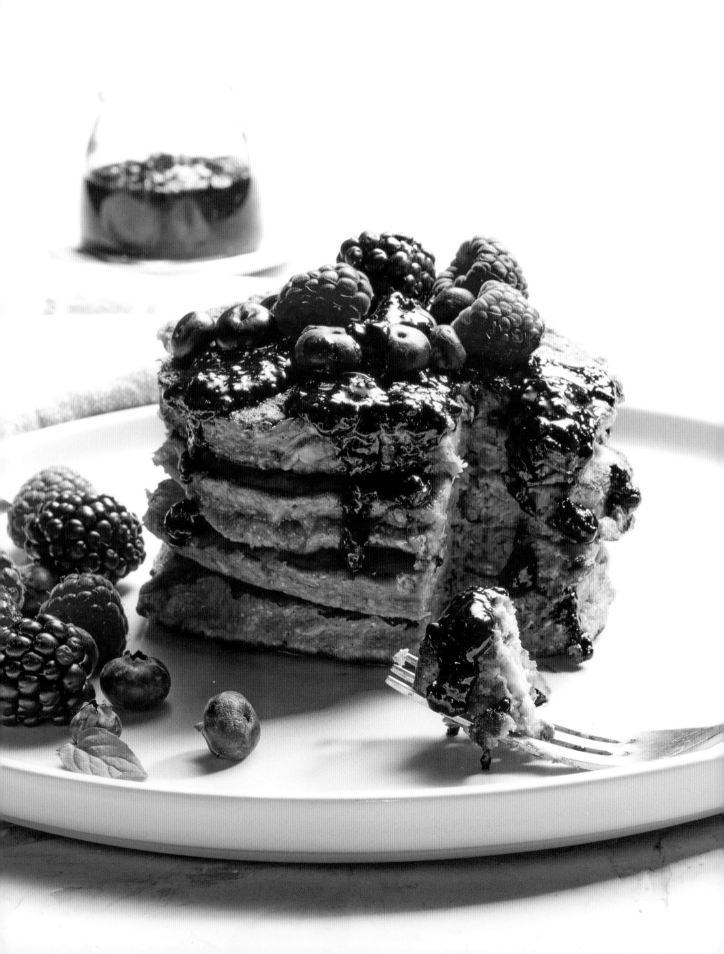

Best Banana Pancakes with Mixed Berry Compote

Makes 4 large pancakes.

These pancakes are so good they don't even need a topping. I usually eat them with just a little melted butter, but I also love them with berries. The compote makes them really special. Feel free to improvise and make your favorite low-carb topping.

Ingredients

Compote

1½ cups mixed berries, fresh or frozen (fully thawed)

1–2 Tbsp. chia seeds

2 tsp. lemon juice

1 tsp. vanilla

Pinch of salt

1 Tbsp. real maple syrup (not pancake syrup) or honey (optional)

Pancakes

2 ripe bananas, mashed

4 whole eggs

½ cup rolled oats

½ cup chickpea flour

1 tsp. vanilla

1 tsp. cinnamon

Pinch of salt

1–2 Tbsp. coconut oil or butter, plus more melted butter for serving

Directions

Compote

Place all ingredients in a blender or food processor and pulse gently until the berries are just combined. Leave them still chunky, so your sauce will have some texture.

Start with just 1 Tbsp. of chia seeds. Use more if needed to soak up the juices. The chia seeds will absorb some of the extra juice and add protein and fiber to balance out the the fruit-based carbohydrates. Taste the compote; if you want it sweeter, add optional maple syrup or honey. Set aside.

Pancakes

Put the mashed bananas into a medium-sized mixing bowl. Add eggs, oats, chickpea flour, vanilla, cinnamon, and salt. Stir until just blended.

Using medium-low heat, warm a sauté pan with butter or coconut oil. When the oil starts to sizzle, pour a quarter of the mixture into the pan. When the pancake starts to bubble on top, turn it over and cook until it's light brown on both sides. Remove it to a plate in a slightly warm oven. Repeat with remaining batter.

Serve with warm melted butter and/or top with the **Mixed Berry Compote.**

Variation

For blueberry pancakes, add fresh or frozen blueberries to the batter before cooking. (If using frozen, be sure the berries are at room temperature. Remove any liquid—you can add it to the compote.)

Protein Porridge with Chia and Quinoa

Makes 4 servings.

Liven up your morning oatmeal by adding more protein and fiber — it will keep you feeling satisfied (and your blood sugar stable) for hours!

Ingredients

- 3 cups milk (any type of dairy or unsweetened non-dairy milk)
- 1 cup gluten-free rolled oats or quinoa flakes (see notes)
- ¼ cup chia seeds
- 2 Tbsp. quinoa
- ½ tsp. cinnamon, plus more for garnish
- ⅛ tsp. salt
- 1 mashed banana

Optional garnishes

- Chopped nuts, to taste
- Sprinkle of cinnamon
- Fresh berries

Directions

Add all ingredients, except the banana, to a saucepan over medium heat and allow to simmer until the quinoa are cooked.

Remove from heat and sweeten, to taste, with the banana. Serve topped with chopped nuts and a sprinkle of cinnamon and/or berries.

Notes

- Not all oats are gluten-free. If you have a sensitivity to gluten, make sure you use oats that are labeled "gluten-free."
- Too much quinoa in this recipe can overpower the flavor. This quantity is just enough to add protein, which along with the fiber in the chia, can slow down any blood sugar spiking.

Variations

You can add chopped nuts, seeds, or unsweetened fresh or dried fruit (e.g., dates, raisins, cranberries, or goji berries) to make a hearty meal.

Easy Cauliflower Quiche Breakfast Muffins

Makes 8 muffins.

These are simple to make. You can prepare them in advance, and store them in the fridge for a quick, convenient breakfast or snack. Just reheat, as needed.

Ingredients

Oil or butter, divided

4 oz. pancetta or bacon, cut into pieces (optional for vegetarians)

½ cup sliced mushrooms, canned or fresh

2 cups riced cauliflower (see note)

1 cup shredded mozzarella cheese

1 cup shredded sharp cheddar cheese

3 large eggs

1 Tbsp. flax seed, freshly ground in a blender, food processor, or coffee grinder

¼ tsp. salt

¼ tsp. chili powder

⅛ tsp. black pepper

Directions

Preheat the oven to 375°F. Coat 8 spaces in a muffin/cupcake tray with oil or butter. Or, to keep cleanup simple, use paper baking cups.

Sauté the pancetta, or bacon, in a pan until you reach the desired level of doneness. (A little crispy is nice.) If using fresh mushrooms, you can add these to the pan for a few minutes at the end to soften them before baking. (If using canned mushrooms, wait to add with other ingredients.)

Drain any oil from the meat and fresh mushrooms, then add to a bowl. Mix in all the other ingredients.

Fill 8 sections of the prepared muffin tray evenly with the mixture.

Bake 30–35 minutes.

Note

The easiest option for this recipe is to use frozen, prepared cauliflower rice that is completely thawed and drained of extra liquid. Alternatively, you can easily make your own with a food processor. If you use fresh cauliflower, add it to the pan with the mushrooms to soften before baking. If you don't like cauliflower, you can use 2 cups of grated zucchini. Squeeze out excess water from the grated zucchini before adding to the mixture.

Variation

Vegetarians can adapt this recipe by just omitting the pancetta or substituting vegetarian sausage crumbles.

Egg Florentine Good Morning Muffins

Makes 8 muffins.

This is a great "make-ahead" breakfast recipe to greet the new day without much effort. They are also impressive to serve to guests for a weekend brunch.

Ingredients

Coconut oil or butter, divided

8–10 slices prosciutto (or sliced ham or turkey bacon)

1 small or ½ a large onion, finely diced

1 4-oz. can sliced mushrooms (or use ½ cup fresh mushroom slices)

1 10-oz. package frozen spinach, defrosted and drained of excess liquid

½ tsp. paprika

¼ tsp. chili powder

¼ tsp. salt, to taste

⅛ tsp. black pepper

1 cup shredded cheese (any kind), divided

4 eggs

1 Tbsp. cream, coconut or dairy

1 medium tomato, diced

Optional garnish

Salsa, to taste

Directions

Preheat oven to 350°F. Coat 8–10 spaces in a deep muffin/cupcake tray with oil or butter.

Use 1 slice of prosciutto to line each of the cups, with the meat sitting on the bottom of the cup and going up the sides. Do not leave any gaps exposing the metal of cups. Set aside.

In a sauté pan, over medium-high heat, add a little coconut oil or butter and then add the onion. Heat and stir until the onion is transparent and soft. Add the mushrooms, spinach, and spices. Heat until well-combined and any excess liquid from the spinach has evaporated.

Remove from heat and mix in ¾ cup of grated cheese. Take a spoonful of the mixture and fill each of the meat-lined cups in the baking tray about halfway.

In a separate bowl, whisk the eggs with the cream and divide evenly among the 8–10 portions to almost fill the wells in the baking tray. Add the diced tomato and remaining cheese on top.

Bake for about 25 minutes, until the muffins do not jiggle, and the cheese is nicely melted. Serve with a dollop of salsa.

Note

Store extra muffins in the refrigerator for up to 3 days to reheat when desired.

Variations

You can also add a variety of your favorite goodies into the mixture. Try pork, turkey, or vegetarian sausage, peppers, garlic, feta, steamed broccoli, fresh parsley or other herbs, and any vegetables you'd like. (Be sure to sauté the vegetables, so you get rid of as much water as possible before mixing in with the eggs.) **Marinated Mushrooms** (see page 108) would also be a great enhancement to this recipe.

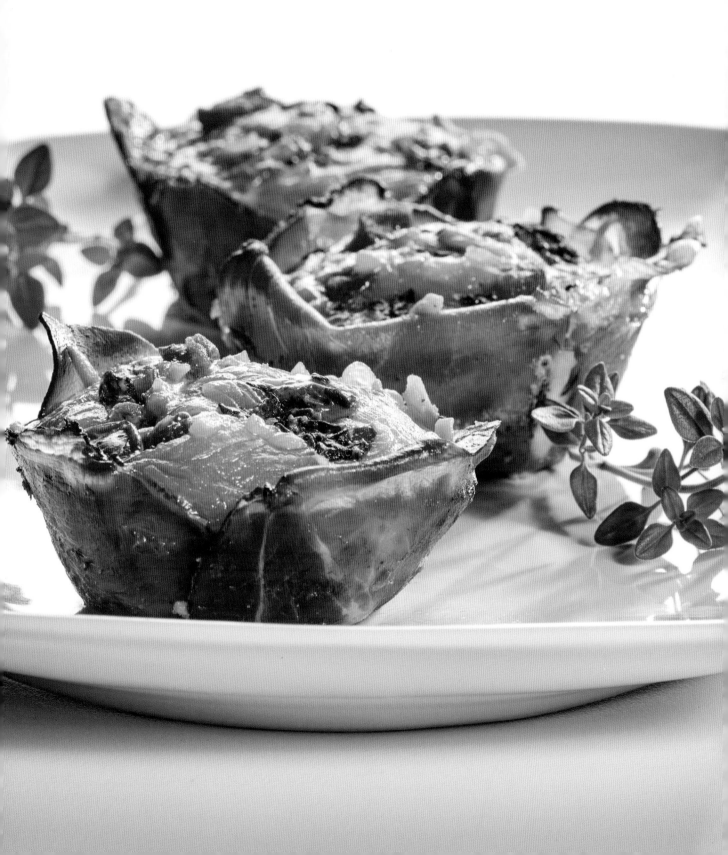

Fried Eggs with Avocado on Sweet Potato "Toast"

Makes 4 servings.

Who doesn't love avocado toast? Did you think you had to give this up just because of diabetes? Here's a delicious version using a slice of sweet potato as your "bread."

Ingredients

- 1 large sweet potato, cleaned and cut lengthwise into 4 even slices, about ¼" thick
- 1 Tbsp. coconut or avocado oil
- 1 avocado
- 1 tsp. lime juice
- ¼ tsp. salt
- ¼ tsp. chili powder
- Dash of black pepper
- 1 tsp. pesto; or make **Basil Pesto Sauce** (see page 74)
- ¼ cup feta cheese
- 4 eggs
- Pat of butter

Directions

Preheat the oven to 400°F. Line a baking sheet with parchment paper.

Place the slices of sweet potato on the baking sheet and brush both sides with oil. Bake in the oven for about 15 minutes on one side, and then flip for another 15 minutes on the other side.

While the sweet potatoes are cooking, mash the avocado in a bowl along with the lime juice, salt, chili powder, pepper, and pesto. Mix in the feta cheese. Set aside.

Fry the eggs in a sauté pan with a little butter. When the sweet potatoes are done, spread the avocado mixture onto each of the sweet potato slices and top with a fried egg.

Variations

Try some fresh herbs like cilantro, basil, or parsley instead of the pesto.

Hearty Sweet Potato, Black Bean, and Egg Burrito

Makes 4 servings.

A lower-carb version of this breakfast favorite that you can enjoy any time of the day.

Ingredients

Spice mix
½ tsp. chili powder

½ tsp. cumin powder

½ tsp. paprika

½ tsp. salt

¼ tsp. black pepper

¼ tsp. garlic powder

¼ tsp. onion powder

Sweet potatoes
4 medium sweet potatoes

For assembly
1–2 Tbsp. butter

2–3 eggs

4 low-carb tortillas or wraps;
or make **Herbed Tortilla Wraps**
(see page 100)

1 15.5-oz. can black beans, drained, rinsed,
and warmed

Optional garnishes
Salsa or hot sauce, to taste

Avocado, diced, to taste

Directions

Preheat the oven to 425°F. Line a baking tray with parchment paper.

Spice mix
Add all the spices together in a bowl and mix thoroughly. Set aside.

Sweet potatoes
Thoroughly wash and dry the sweet potatoes. Use a fork or a knife to poke holes in each potato to let steam escape while cooking. Bake the sweet potatoes for 45–60 minutes on your prepared tray. A fork or knife will insert easily into the center of a potato when it has finished baking.

Remove the sweet potatoes from the oven and allow them to cool for a few minutes. Cut in half, lengthwise; scoop out the soft inner flesh and place it in a bowl. Start with 2 tsp. of spice mixture (about ½ tsp. per potato, if scaling) and mash together until evenly distributed. Taste to ensure the flavor is to your liking. Add more spice, if desired. Set aside.

Assemble
Add a little butter to a sauté pan and scramble the eggs over medium heat. Remove eggs from pan and set aside.

Warm a tortilla briefly in the sauté pan. After it is heated, move to a plate.

Spread a generous spoonful of the sweet potato mash onto the tortilla wrap, add a scoop of heated black beans and ¼ of the scrambled eggs. Roll the tortilla. Repeat with the other three wraps. Serve with a little salsa and avocado on the side.

Note
Pre-mix spices in bulk and store any extra spice mix in a sealed glass container. Use whenever you need a delicious spice mix to conveniently season a savory meal.

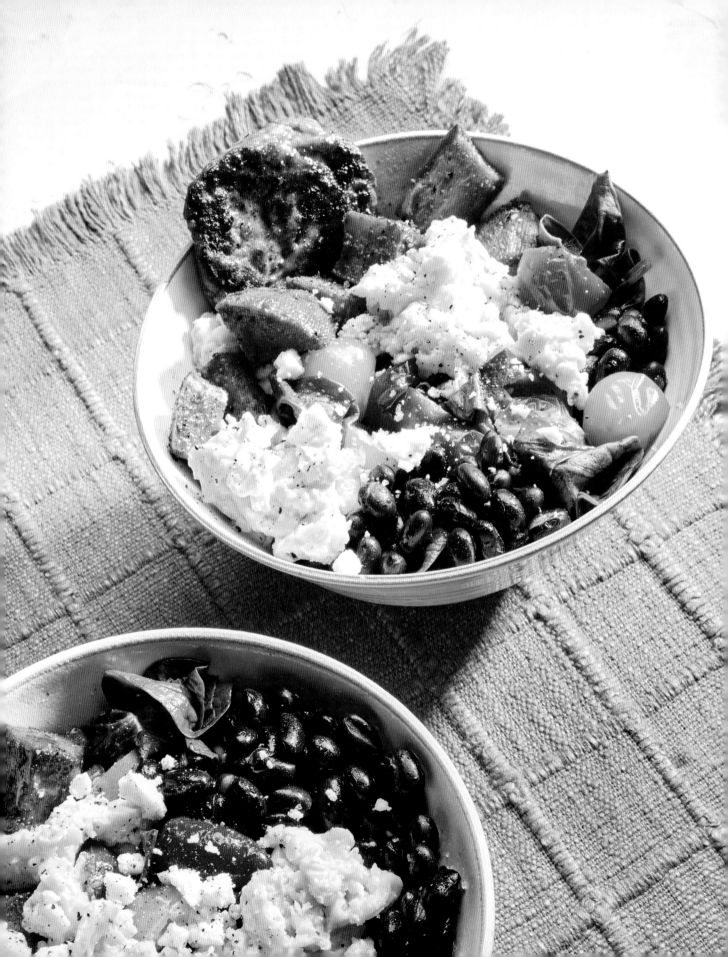

Bountiful Breakfast Bowl

Makes 4 bowls.

This is a great breakfast or brunch item when you have time to relax and enjoy a filling meal.

Ingredients

Sweet potato cubes

2-3 sweet potatoes, peeled and cut into 1" cubes

2 Tbsp. avocado oil

½ tsp. cumin

½ tsp. garlic powder

½ tsp. paprika

Salt and black pepper, to taste

Bowl

2 Tbsp. coconut or avocado oil

2 small cloves garlic, minced

2-3 cups spinach or kale

1 cup cherry tomatoes, halved

1-3 tsp. water

1 15-oz. can black beans, rinsed and drained

8 oz. pre-cooked breakfast sausage (optional)

4-6 eggs (scrambled or prepared according to your preference)

Salt and pepper, to taste

Optional garnishes

Feta or cotija cheese, to taste

Fresh herbs, like cilantro, parsley, etc.

1 avocado, sliced

Hot sauce or lime juice, to taste

Directions

Preheat oven to 425°F. Line a baking tray with parchment paper.

Sweet potato cubes

Toss the potatoes with avocado oil and spices, making sure they're mixed well. Arrange the sweet potato cubes in a single layer on the baking sheet. Roast in the oven for 30–35 minutes. Stir the potatoes halfway through to ensure all sides are cooked thoroughly.

Bowl

While the potatoes are roasting, prepare the vegetables. In a small skillet, heat oil over medium heat. Add garlic; cook 30 seconds. Add spinach or kale, tomatoes, and a bit of the water, if needed, to wilt the greens. Cook, stirring often, until softened, 2 to 3 minutes. Remove from heat and set aside on a plate.

Add the black beans (and sausage, if using) to the same skillet, without cleaning it. Heat until browned, about 2 minutes. Set aside, covered, to keep warm.

Cook eggs to your desired preference—scrambled is easy, but anything will work.

Assemble

Scoop a little bit of each of the ingredients into four bowls: roasted sweet potato cubes, greens with tomatoes, black beans (with sausage), and eggs. Season with salt and black pepper.

Garnish with cheese, fresh herbs, and/or avocado, if desired. Serve warm with a few dashes of hot sauce or lime juice, if that is your preference.

Note

Sweet potato cubes can be roasted in advance or the night before to save time. Reheat when ready to assemble.

Guacamole Breakfast Sandwich

Makes 4 sandwiches.

A filling and delicious treat to start your day, plus you won't have to worry about carbs. Wow!

Ingredients

4 slices bacon or 4 sausage patties (optional)

1–2 Tbsp. butter, divided

Mushrooms and/or roasted red pepper, sliced

8 eggs

Splash of milk or coconut cream

Salt and black pepper, to taste

4 low-carb burger buns; or make **(You Don't Need a Lettuce Wrap) Burger Buns** (see page 105)

½ cup sharp cheddar or mozzarella cheese

Sauce of your choice; or make **Spicy Garlic Tomato Sauce** (see page 111) and/or **Basil Pesto Sauce** (see recipe page 74)

½ cup guacamole; or make **Easy Guacamole** (see page 115)

Directions

If using meat, cook according to directions on the package. Set aside.

Using a small amount of butter, fry up some sliced mushrooms and/or roasted red peppers in a pan. Let rest while you scramble the eggs, using the eggs, milk and salt and pepper.

To assemble your sandwiches, start by slicing the burger buns in half and toasting them. Then build your sandwich on the bottom bun. Start with a layer of cheese. Next, put on the bacon or sausage and eggs. Add the **Spicy Garlic Tomato Sauce** or **Basil Pesto** and a scoop of **Easy Guacamole.** Toss on the prepared mushrooms/peppers. Finally, close the sandwich with the top bun.

Note

Prepared roasted red pepper slices are easily sourced. They are commonly found in a glass jar in the condiment aisle of your grocery store.

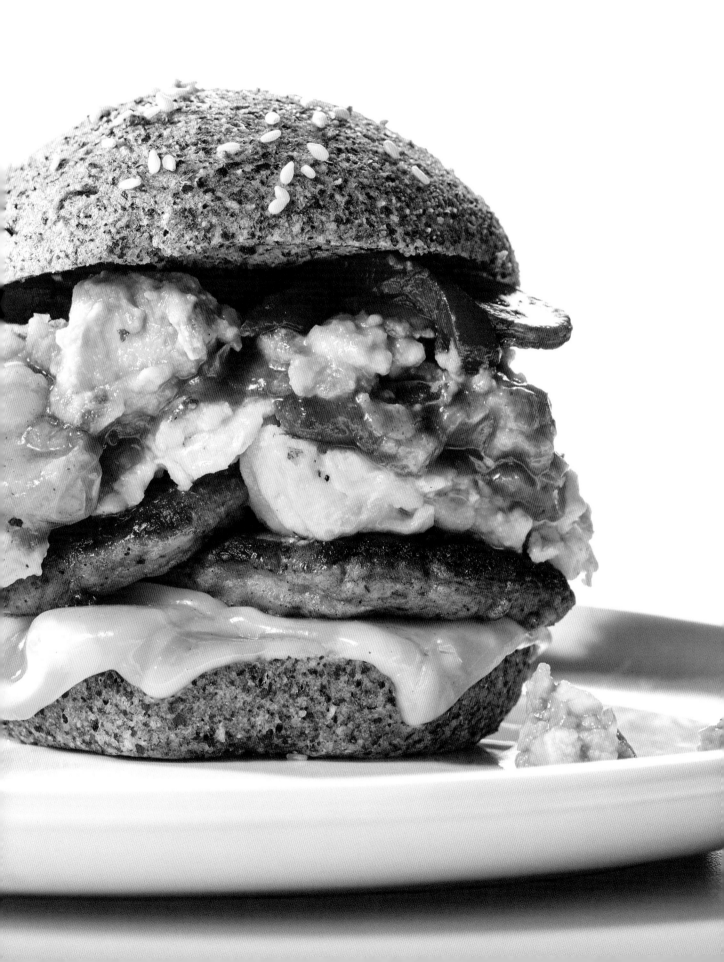

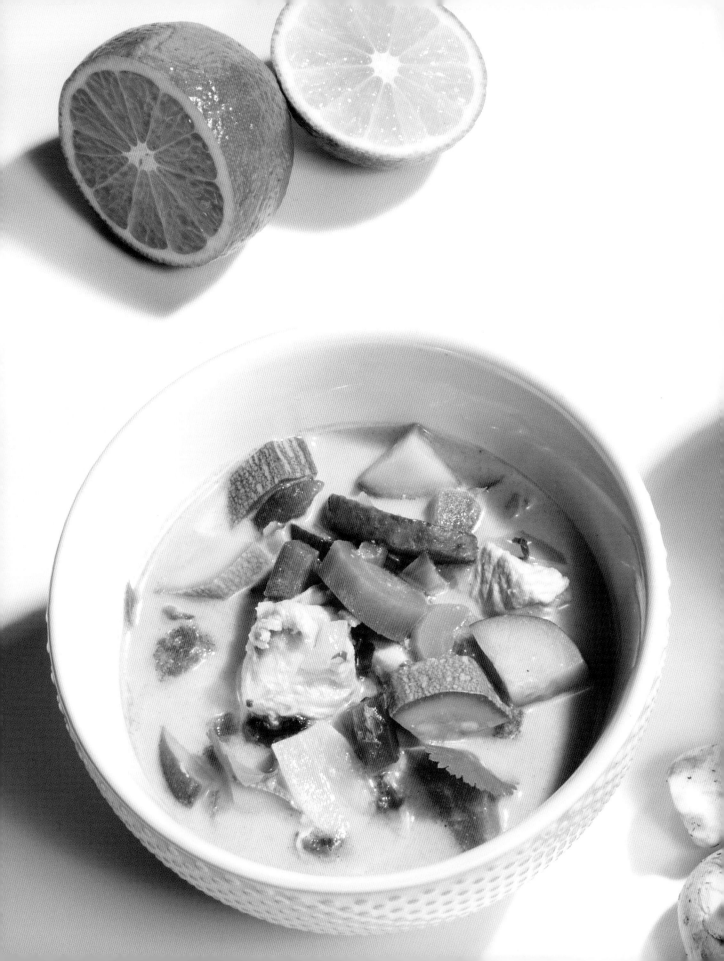

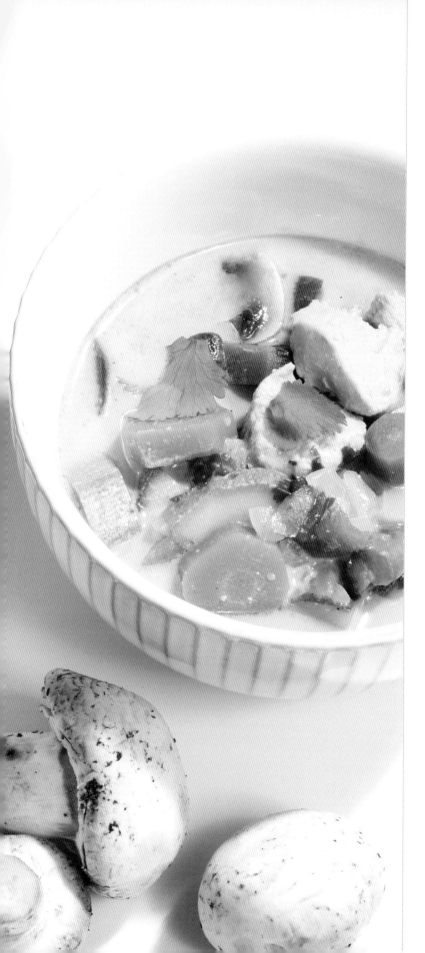

SOUPS & STEWS

Immune-Boosting Detox Vegetable Soup

Makes 4–6 servings.

This is one of my go-to healthy favorites and is filling enough for a lunch. It is a regular in my food prep schedule.

Ingredients

1 Tbsp. coconut oil or avocado oil

1 large onion, diced

1 quart of your favorite stock or broth

4–5 stalks celery, chopped

1 fennel bulb, chopped

1 small head of broccoli, chopped

1 bunch asparagus, trimmed and chopped

1 zucchini, chopped

5 dinosaur (lacinato) kale leaves, chopped

Water

½ cup coconut cream

Small handful fresh cilantro (optional)

Small handful fresh parsley (optional)

2–3 tsp. freshly grated ginger root

3 large cloves garlic, minced

Juice of 1 lemon or 2 limes

1½ tsp. salt

1 tsp. cumin

½ tsp. chili powder

⅛ tsp. cayenne pepper

Optional garnishes

Pumpkin seeds, to taste

Avocado diced, to taste

Directions

In a large soup pot on medium heat, add oil and onions. Sauté until the onions soften. Stir in the other vegetables and the stock, adding additional water, if needed, to just cover the vegetables in the pot.

Bring the contents to a boil. Then turn down the heat and simmer, covered, approximately 20 minutes—until vegetables are soft.

In a blender, add the coconut cream, cilantro, parsley, ginger, garlic, lemon/lime, and spices. Blend until creamy, or until there are just flecks of the green herbs in the mixture. After the vegetables have simmered, add the cream mixture to the pot and stir to combine.

If you'd like a smooth texture, you can put some of the soup, in small batches, back into the blender to break into smaller pieces. Leave it a little chunky for the best texture.

When you have created the consistency you like, taste and adjust for final flavor balance. Serve as is or garnish with seasoned pumpkin seeds and/or avocado chunks for a heartier soup.

Variation

If you don't have one or two of the vegetables this recipe calls for, don't worry—you can use a collection of any green vegetables (pick 3–5 of your favorites), in addition to the onion base.

Green vegetables, and leafy greens in particular, are some of the most important foods that should be included in your daily diet. The benefits are incredible. Greens are low in calories, high in fiber, vitamins, and phytonutrients.

Getting a variety of greens is important – there are many greens to choose from, so switch it up! Try kale, spinach, collard greens, broccoli, broccoli sprouts, cabbage, beet greens, watercress, arugula, mustard greens, Swiss chard, bok choy, or romaine lettuce.

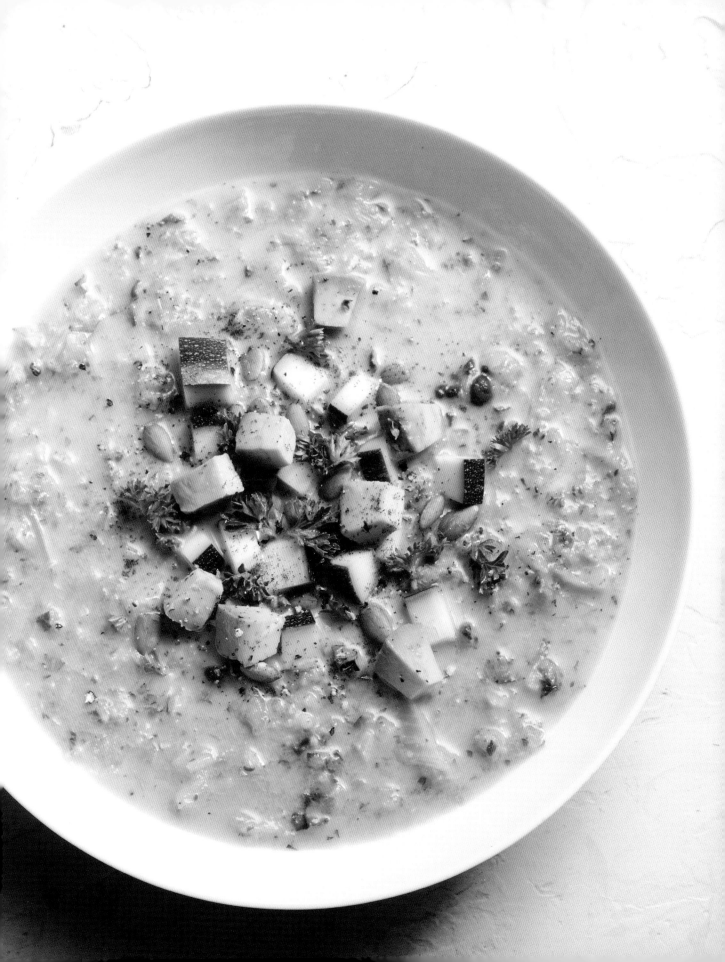

Sweet Potato Lentil Chili

Makes 6–8 servings.

For chili lovers — you'll never miss the meat!

Ingredients

1–2 Tbsp. avocado or coconut oil

2 medium onions, diced

1 cup celery, diced

3 sweet potatoes, peeled and cut into 1" cubes

3 large cloves garlic, minced

1½ tsp. salt

Black pepper, to taste

2 tsp. chili powder

1 tsp. cumin

1 tsp. paprika

½ tsp. freshly grated nutmeg, or nutmeg powder

½ tsp. crushed red pepper flakes (or to taste)

¼ tsp. cinnamon

¼ tsp. cayenne pepper (optional, if you like spicy)

1 quart vegetable broth, your favorite stock, or water

1 28-oz. can crushed tomatoes

1 14-oz. can black beans, rinsed

1 14-oz. can kidney beans, rinsed

1½ cups dry red lentils

3 Tbsp. freshly-squeezed lime juice

Optional garnishes

Avocado chunks

Sour cream; or make **Cashew Sour Cream** (see page 109), to taste

Directions

To a large pot on medium heat, add oil and onions. Sauté until the onions soften. Add celery, sweet potatoes, garlic, salt, pepper, and spices. Stir thoroughly. Add the broth or liquid, tomatoes, beans, and lentils.

Increase heat and bring to a boil. Then reduce the heat and simmer for about 25 minutes, or until the sweet potatoes are softened, stirring occasionally. Add in lime juice at the end and taste to adjust spices.

Serve with avocado chucks and a dollop of sour cream or **Cashew Sour Cream.**

Variation

Roast the sweet potato cubes before adding to the pot, for a richer flavor.

Serving suggestion

Serve with **Chickpea Veggie Skillet Bread**.

White Bean & Kale Stew with Roasted Squash

Makes 4-6 servings.

Rich and hearty, this stew is chock full of fiber and nutrition. It's excellent comfort food!

Ingredients

14 oz. (3-4 cups) butternut squash, cut into small cubes

3 Tbsp. coconut or avocado oil, divided

2 tsp. salt, divided

½ tsp. black pepper, divided

2 medium leeks, cleaned and chopped, white and light green parts only

½ tsp. rosemary

1 15-oz. can white cannellini beans (or 1½ cups of any cooked, white bean), drained and rinsed

4-5 cups kale, cut into thin strips

3 stalks celery, sliced

2-3 medium carrots, sliced or diced

2-3 diced tomatoes with juice (or 1 15-oz. can)

3 large cloves garlic, minced

2 cups vegetable broth

2½ tsp. apple cider vinegar

1 tsp. thyme

1 tsp. crushed red pepper

1 pinch cayenne pepper

Directions

Preheat oven to 425°F. Line a baking tray with parchment paper.

Place squash in a mixing bowl. Drizzle with oil and season with ½ tsp. salt and ¼ tsp. black pepper. Mix to combine, then transfer to the prepared tray. Spread the squash out and roast in the oven, stirring occasionally for 25–30 minutes until squash is tender and caramelized at the edges.

While the squash is roasting, warm the rest of the oil in a large soup pot, on medium heat. Add the sliced/chopped leeks, rosemary, and ½ tsp. salt. Cook, stirring occasionally so the leeks won't burn, about 10–15 minutes.

Add the beans, kale, celery, carrots, tomato, garlic, and broth and simmer for 10–15 minutes, until the vegetables are tender. When the vegetables are cooked through, add the roasted squash.

Season with the apple cider vinegar, the remaining salt, thyme, and crushed red pepper. Taste and adjust the salt, black pepper, and cayenne pepper to your liking.

Note

If you are in a hurry, you can omit the roasting step. Just add the squash directly into the pan with the beans and other vegetables. It won't be quite as flavorful, but will save time.

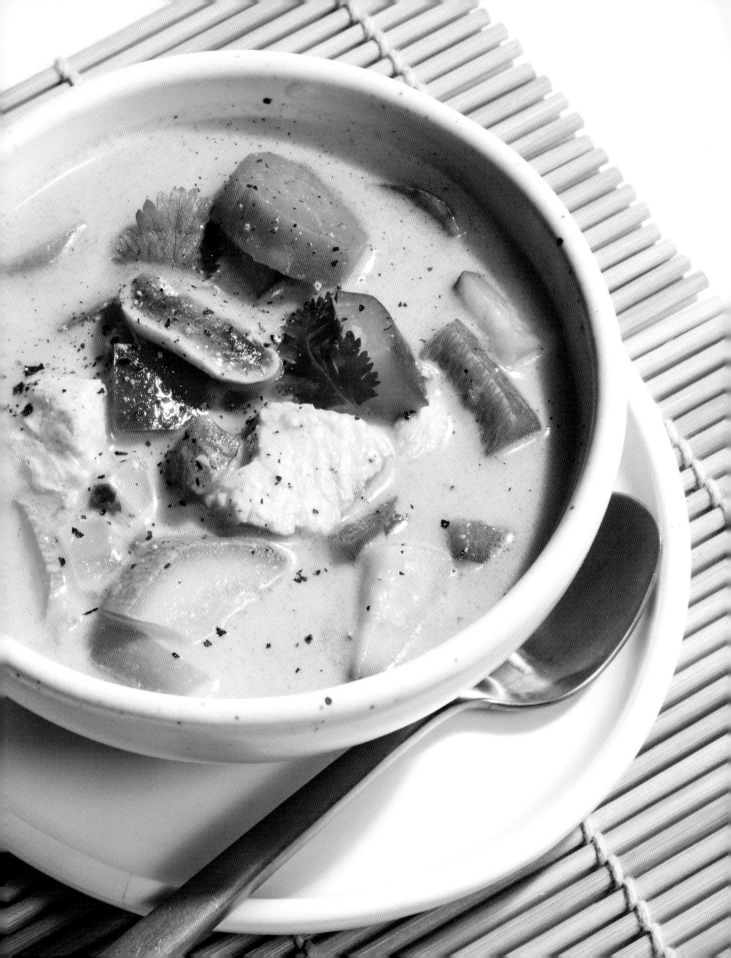

Coconut & Lime Chicken Soup

Makes 4–6 servings.

A light and tangy soup that will soon be a family favorite!

Ingredients

2–3 Tbsp. coconut oil or avocado oil

1 lb. boneless, skinless chicken breast, cut into bite-sized pieces

1 medium or large onion, finely diced

3 cloves garlic, minced

2–3 tsp. fresh ginger, finely minced

1 medium tomato, diced

1 medium carrot, grated or finely diced

½–1 bell pepper, seeds removed, finely diced

½ cup sliced mushrooms, fresh or canned

1 quart chicken broth

1 medium zucchini, diced

⅔ cup coconut cream or 1 13-oz. can coconut milk

¼ cup fresh cilantro, parsley or other herbs, finely chopped

Juice of 1 lime

2 tsp. salt, or to taste

½ tsp. black pepper, or to taste

Directions

In a large soup pot, add the oil, chicken, and onion. Sauté over medium-high heat until the onion begins to soften and the chicken is no longer pink — about 5 minutes. Stir intermittently.

Add the garlic, ginger, and remaining vegetables, except the herbs and zucchini. Heat for 1–2 minutes, stirring to combine all the ingredients together.

Add the chicken broth and zucchini and bring to a boil. Then, reduce heat and simmer for about 15 minutes, until the vegetables are soft.

Add the coconut milk or cream, herbs, lime juice, salt and pepper. Taste and adjust the flavors. Serve hot.

Note

You can use shredded, pre-cooked rotisserie chicken to save time. Add it in with the zucchini.

Lemon Fennel Soup with White Beans Topped with Roasted Brussels Sprouts

Makes 4-6 servings.

Try not to eat all the roasted brussels sprouts leaves before you garnish — I dare you!

Ingredients

Soup

    2 Tbsp. coconut or avocado oil
    1 large yellow onion, sliced
    ½ tsp. fennel seeds, coarsely ground
    3 cloves garlic, minced
½–1 tsp. salt
    Dash of cayenne pepper
    1 15-oz. can of white beans,
      rinsed and drained
    1 fennel bulb, sliced
    1 quart chicken or vegetable stock
    Juice of 1 lemon, divided
    Shredded, pre-cooked chicken (optional)

Topping

    10–15 brussels sprouts, leaves separated
    Drizzle of avocado oil
    Juice from half a lemon
    Salt and black pepper, to taste

Directions

Pre-heat the oven to 350°F.

Soup

Heat the oil in a large saucepan over medium heat. Add the onion and the fennel seed. Cook until the onion is soft and starting to brown. Add the garlic, salt, and pepper and heat for another two minutes, stirring periodically.

Add the white beans, sliced fennel, and broth. Bring to a boil, then reduce to a simmer. Cover and cook for about 20–30 minutes.

Add juice from half a lemon to the cooked soup. Using either a standard blender or an immersion blender, blend the soup until smooth. After the soup is puréed, add the shredded chicken (if using) to the soup for protein and texture. Taste and adjust seasoning.

Topping

Spread the leaves out evenly onto a baking sheet, drizzle with avocado oil and lemon juice. Season with salt and pepper. Give them a gentle toss to coat. Roast in the oven, until they are crispy and the edges start to brown, about 8–10 minutes.

Assemble

Ladle the soup into bowls. Top with a handful of the crispy brussels sprouts leaves and serve immediately. The sprouts are best enjoyed hot and fresh from the oven.

Note

Prepare the brussels sprouts leaves while the soup is simmering. Or, if you're in a hurry, you could leave off the brussels sprouts topping. You'll still have a delicious meal.

Everyone Loves Chili

Makes 6-8 servings.

Although this recipe will appeal to meat lovers, vegetarians can omit the meat and use more varieties of beans instead. Perfect meal before watching your favorite sport on TV.

Ingredients

- 1 Tbsp. coconut or avocado oil
- 1 lb. ground beef (or bison)
- 1 onion, chopped
- 1 large carrot, grated
- 3 celery stalks, chopped
- 1 bell pepper, seeded and diced
- 1 zucchini, diced
- 2 cups water or your favorite stock
- 1 28-oz. can crushed tomatoes (including liquid)
- 1 15-oz. can kidney beans, rinsed and drained (or any beans you like)
- 1 15-oz. can black beans, rinsed and drained (or any beans you like)
- 2-3 Tbsp. tomato paste
- 2-3 tsp. garlic, minced (4-5 cloves)
- 2 Tbsp. chili powder
- 1 tsp. cumin
- 1 tsp. salt
- 1 tsp. dried oregano or Italian herbs
- ½ tsp. smoked paprika
- ½ tsp. black pepper
- ½ cup coconut cream
- Juice of 1 lime

Optional garnishes

- 1 avocado, peeled, pitted, and diced
- Small handful fresh cilantro, chopped
- Sprinkle of minced jalapeno
- Sprinkle of cayenne pepper

Directions

Warm the oil in a large pot over medium heat. Place the ground beef in the pot and cook until evenly browned.

Stir in onion, carrot, celery, bell pepper, and zucchini. Pour water or stock into the pot. Add the tomatoes, beans, and tomato paste. Season with garlic, chili powder, cumin, salt, oregano, paprika, and pepper. Bring to a boil. Reduce heat to low, cover, and simmer 15-25 minutes to soften the vegetables and thicken the chili. Stir in the coconut cream and add the lime juice at the end.

Pour into bowls and garnish with avocado chunks and chopped cilantro. If you like a spicy chili, add some jalapeno and/or cayenne pepper.

Note

Coconut cream adds a comfort factor, while keeping the recipe dairy-free. You can substitute a dollop of sour cream for the coconut cream in the recipe, if desired.

Variations

If you don't want to use beef or bison, you can swap it with ground turkey or chopped chicken breasts. Or, you can leave out the meat entirely. Add 1½ cups cooked lentils or chickpeas instead—red lentils are my favorite!

Serving suggestions

This would go well with the **Chickpea Veggie Skillet Bread** (see page 101), **Herbed Rolls** (see page 102), or **Herbed Tortilla Wraps** (see page 100).

Moroccan Beef Stew

Makes 6–8 servings.

Impress your friends with this dish. Serve it along with some grain-free pita bread, extra virgin olive oil with spices for dipping, and a small bowl of olives. You'll have plenty of food for conversation!

Ingredients

- 1 lb. chuck roast or brisket (stew meat)
- 2 Tbsp. coconut oil or avocado oil
- 1 onion, diced
- 1 Tbsp. chickpea flour
- ½ Tbsp. fresh ginger (about 1" of ginger), finely grated or 1 tsp. ginger powder
- 4 tsp. fresh garlic, minced
- 1½ tsp. sweet paprika or smoked paprika
- 1½ tsp. salt
- 1 tsp. cinnamon
- 1 tsp. coriander
- ½ tsp. turmeric
- ½ tsp. cumin
- ½ tsp. crushed red pepper
- ¼ tsp. black pepper
- 2 Tbsp. tomato paste
- 1 quart beef stock (or water)
- ½ cup medjool dates (about 8–10), pits removed and diced
- 2 medium carrots, diced
- 1 28-oz. can diced tomatoes
- 1 15-oz. can chickpeas (about 1½ cups cooked)

Optional garnish
- Parsley, to taste

Directions

Cube the meat into 1" squares. In a large stockpot, heat the oil. When hot, add the beef cubes and cook until brown and all the juices have been released. Add the onion and reduce the heat to medium. Cook the onion with the beef for about 5 minutes, until the onion becomes soft.

Add the chickpea flour, ginger, garlic, spices, and tomato paste. Stir well, until everything is mixed and there are no clumps. You will start to notice the fragrance as it cooks. Add a little of the beef broth (or water) to deglaze the pan, then add the rest of the liquid, along with the dates, carrots, tomatoes, and chickpeas.

Bring everything to a boil, then reduce the heat and simmer for 1½–2 hours on very low heat, covered, until the meat is tender.

Taste the gravy and adjust seasoning, as desired.

Add a sprig or two of parsley when dishing into individual bowls.

Note

This stew can be made in a crockpot.

Variation

Medjool dates are my favorite and the easiest to use, but any other dates will work. Or substitute raisins, if necessary, to create a similar effect.

Serving suggestion

Serve this with **Grain-Free Pita Pockets** (see page 98). You can also enjoy it on a bed of **Basic Cauliflower Rice** (see page 108), or with a side dish of steamed green beans or broccoli.

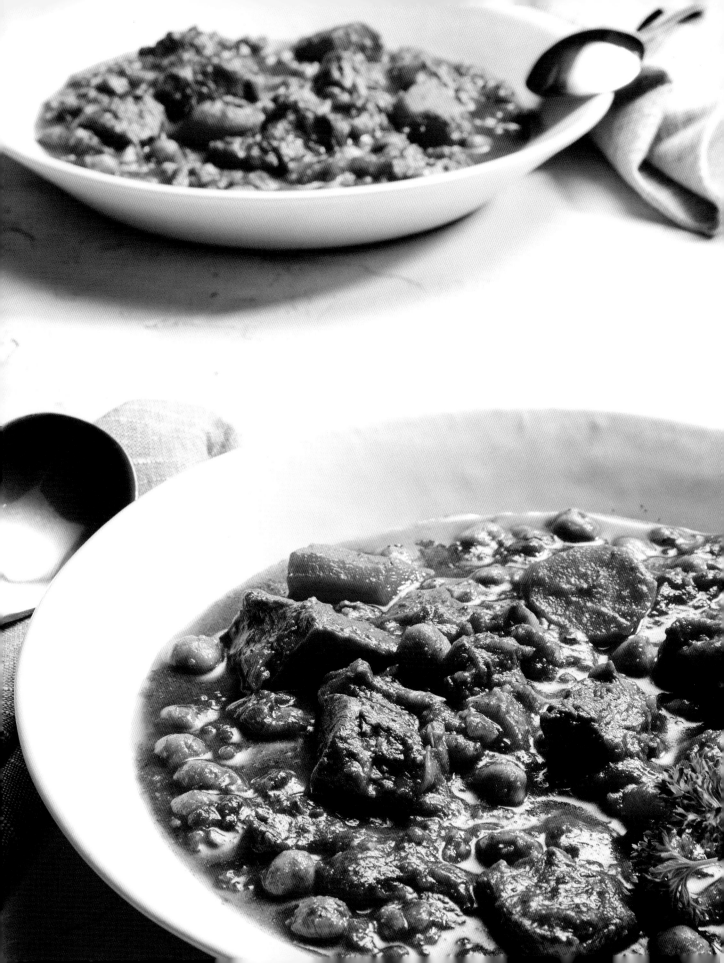

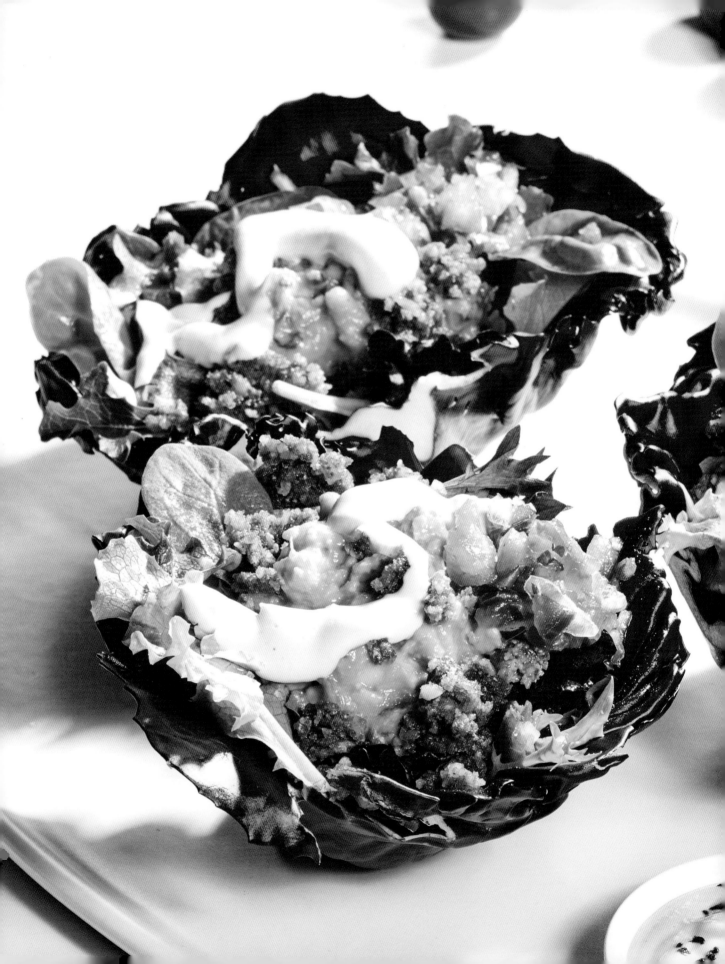

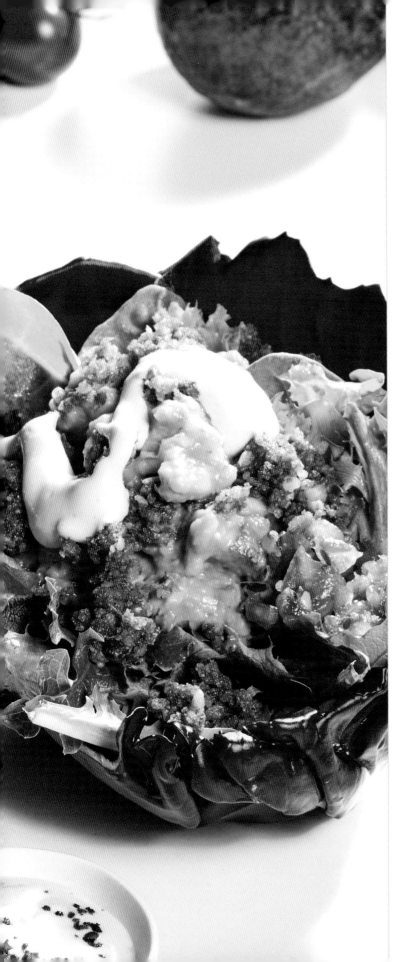

SALADS

Kelp Noodle Salad

Makes 4 servings.

I created this recipe during a visit to Iceland. I served it to our guests for lunch and everyone loved it!

Ingredients

1 12-oz. package kelp noodles
(or substitute zucchini noodles)

½ cup pesto; or make **Basil Pesto Sauce**
(see page 74)

1 avocado, peeled, pitted, and diced

1 cup cherry tomatoes, halved

Feta cheese (optional)

¼ cup olives, pitted and cut in half, to taste

Handful of fresh baby spinach,
cut into ribbons

Optional garnish

Capers, to taste

Directions

Soak the kelp noodles in warm, filtered water for 5 to 10 minutes. Drain the noodles and then cut them into manageable lengths. (If using zucchini noodles, there is no need to soak or heat the zucchini. Keep it raw.)

In a large serving bowl, toss the noodles with the pesto, then add the avocado, tomatoes, feta, and olives. Stir, until everything is evenly coated with pesto.

Mix in the spinach ribbons, then garnish with capers. Serve immediately as either a light entrée or as a side dish.

Serving suggestion

This salad is delicious as a base for the **Mushroom Artichoke Pesto Chicken** (see page 86).

Kelp noodles are, as the name implies, noodles that are made from kelp seaweed. When you look at these clear, thin noodles, you would not know this. They are almost flavorless, so don't be put off by the concern that they might taste fishy.

Kelp noodles take on the flavor of any foods they are paired with, so they are typically used as a grain-free, gluten-free, and nearly calorie-free replacement for pasta, or in stir-frys, salads, or curries. When used raw, they have a nice crunch to them. Cooked, they become very soft.

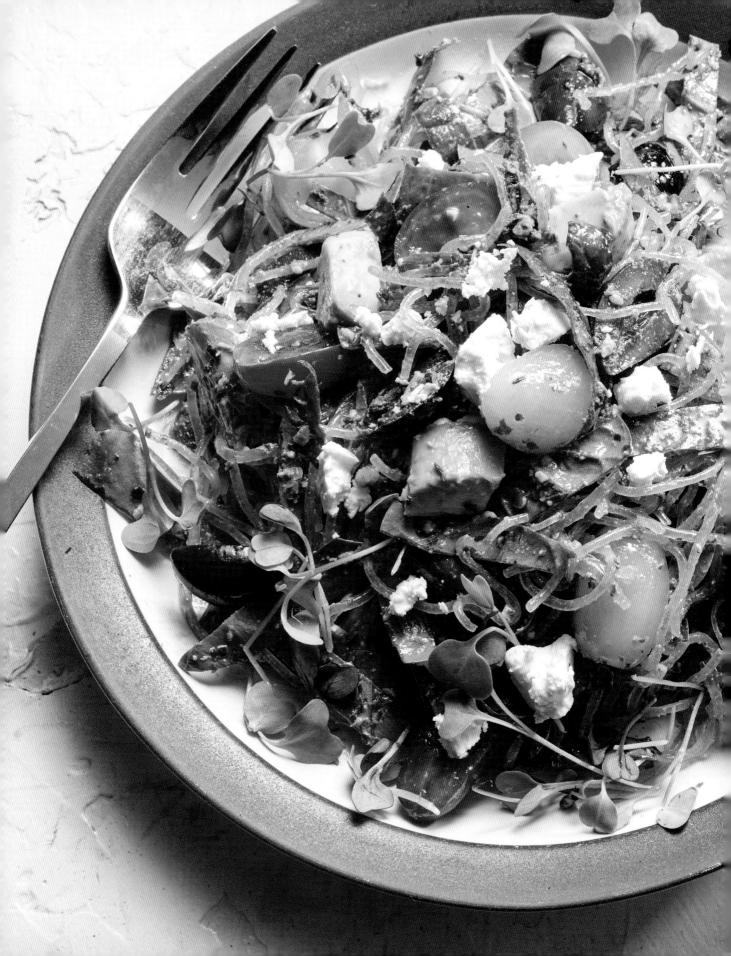

Kale Salad with Pistachios & Cranberries

Makes 4 servings.

This recipe is a classic that I often bring to potlucks or family gatherings and it's always a winner! The juxtaposition of colors, flavors, and textures makes this salad special.

Ingredients

- 1 bunch curly kale
- Juice of one lemon
- 3–4 Tbsp. extra virgin olive oil
- 2–3 tsp. honey, or coconut nectar
- Salt, to taste
- 1 small bulb fennel or ½ cup shredded purple cabbage (optional)
- Shredded carrots (optional)
- Pistachios, to taste
- Dried cranberries, to taste
- Dash of cayenne pepper (optional)

Directions

Separate the kale leaves from the stems and tear or chop the leaves into small, bite-sized pieces. (Curly kale works the best in this recipe, although sometimes I add a little purple kale for color.) Place in a large bowl.

Add lemon, olive oil, sweetener of choice, and salt. Massage the leaves by hand until soft; they should resemble a "cooked" appearance. The acid and salt will further break down the fibers in the kale.

Thinly slice the fennel or cabbage with a food processor, mandoline, or knife and add to the kale. Toss the carrots into the salad and distribute the dressing well.

Garnish with pistachios and dried cranberries. These will add both texture and flavor to the salad.

Variations

You can substitute any nuts and dried fruit for the pistachios and cranberries. Try pecans and dried cherries together, or sliced almonds and chopped dates.

Vegan Tuna Salad

Makes 4 servings.

Vegans and meat lovers alike should try this recipe—it's delicious and filling. You'll love how good it tastes!

Ingredients

Vegan tuna

2 cups raw, unsalted almonds, soaked about 8 hours or overnight, and drained (see notes)

1 sheet nori seaweed, chopped or cut with scissors into small pieces (see notes)

3 stalks celery, diced

3 green onions, sliced thinly

¼ cup lemon juice

1–2 Tbsp. fresh parsley, minced

1 small clove garlic, minced

1 tsp. salt

Dash cayenne pepper

Vegan mayo

1 cup pine nuts

1 large or 2 small avocados, peeled, pitted, and diced

9 dates, pits removed

2 Tbsp. apple cider vinegar

4 tsp. lemon juice

½ clove garlic

1 tsp. salt

Directions

Vegan tuna

Process the almonds and nori in a food processor until finely ground, about 1–2 minutes.

Put ground almonds into a mixing bowl. Add the other Vegan Tuna ingredients and mix until just combined. Set aside while you prepare the mayo.

Vegan mayo

Blend all mayo ingredients together in a food processor, blender, or high-performance blender, until creamy.

Assemble

Add the avocado mayo to the almond mixture and combine. Serve as you might traditional tuna salad—as a filling for a sandwich on your choice of grain-free bread. It would also be tasty as an entrée salad, heaped onto a bed of greens.

Notes

- It's important to use raw almonds in this recipe. Roasted almonds have a different taste and consistency. Plus, when you heat the oils intrinsic to the nut (as in roasting) you create additional toxins that your body must process.

- Some people remove the fibrous husk that comes off the almonds after they have been soaking several hours. This makes for a lighter texture and color in the finished product, but is time consuming and optional.

- Nori sheets can be found in the Asian section of the grocery.

Beyond this recipe

Take a sheet of Nori or a collard green leaf, some of the Vegan Tuna, and chopped vegetables to make a Vegan Tuna cone. Also, you can use this vegan mayo in place of regular mayo in any recipe.

Ajwain seeds are rich in vitamins, minerals, fiber, and antioxidants.
It's interesting to note that in India, Ajwain seeds are known for their
medicinal value, especially in helping digestive problems.
Roasting or toasting ajwain seeds refines the aroma as well as the flavor.

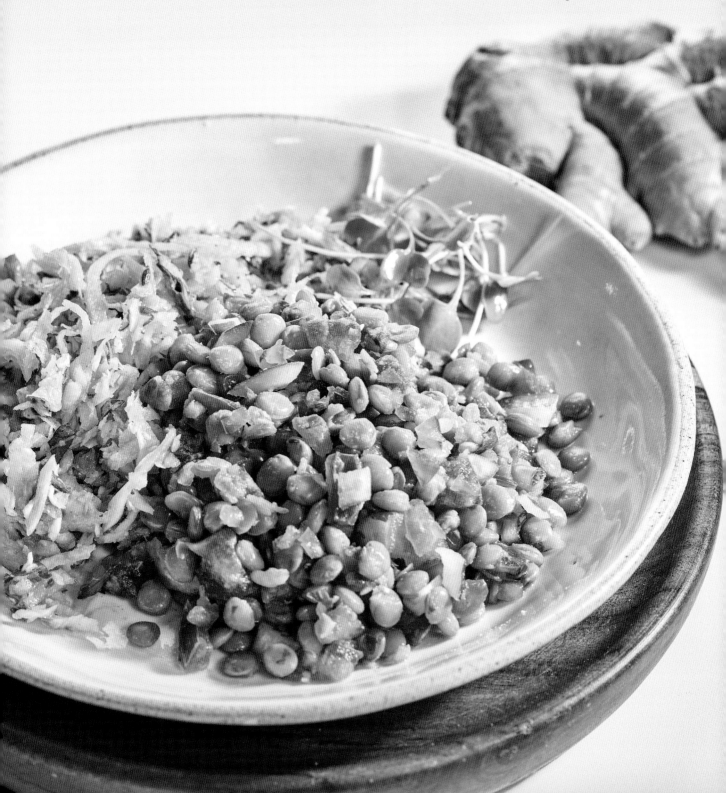

Kitcheree Salad with Lentils

Makes 4–6 servings.

This recipe brings a little taste of India to the western table. The complexity of flavor comes from the layers of spices that Indian culture excels at.

Ingredients

Legumes, part 1

1 cup split mung beans or green lentils

2 cups water or your favorite stock plus water, for soaking

Salad

2 Tbsp. coconut oil, avocado oil, or ghee

¼ tsp. mustard seeds

½ tsp. ajwain seed or carom seed

1 tsp. whole cumin seeds (see note)

1½ cups cabbage, shredded in a food processor using the grater blade, or grated by hand

1 rutabaga, shredded in a food processor using the grater blade, or grated by hand (or substitute turnip or jicama)

½ cup fresh basil leaves, chopped

½ cup fresh cilantro leaves, chopped (optional)

1 tsp. coriander

1 tsp. fresh ginger, finely minced

½ tsp. salt

½ tsp. cumin powder

½ tsp. turmeric

⅛ tsp. cayenne

1 tsp. minced jalapeño (optional)

Splash of olive oil

Legumes, part 2

½ cup pico de gallo, or salsa; or make **Fresh Tomato Salsa** (see page 114)

Directions

Legumes, part 1

Put mung beans or lentils in a medium mixing bowl with enough water to cover them. Let them soak for at least an hour.

Salad

In a sauté pan, add the oil or ghee and heat on medium. When the oil is hot, add the mustard seed, ajwain seed, and cumin seed. Cook briefly to release their fragrance. Be careful not to burn these spices, as this could spoil the taste of the whole dish.

After the spices have heated, add them—along with the oil—to a large mixing bowl with all the other salad ingredients. Mix to combine evenly. Taste and adjust seasoning.

Legumes, part 2

Drain the soaking water from the mung beans (or lentils). Cook them according to directions on the package. (This is usually a 2:1 ratio of liquid to beans. If this is the case, you will use 2 cups of water or stock for the 1 cup of dried beans you started with in Part 1.) Bring to a boil, then reduce heat, and simmer for about 20–25 minutes, depending on which bean you use. When the mung beans (or lentils) have finished cooking, strain any excess water and mix with the salsa.

Assemble

Place a big scoop of the salad mixture on a plate. Add a generous portion of the legumes mixture on top of or beside the salad and serve warm or at room temperature.

Note

While you don't *need* to heat the whole seeds, cooking these spices to release their fragrance before you add them into the salad will give the dish a much richer flavor and taste experience.

Purple Cabbage Vegan Taco Cups

Makes 4 servings.

This salad is very filling and makes a beautiful main course. And, while it may require a bit of work, the result is worth it. Meat lovers will be astounded and never miss the ground beef that is not present. Try it—you'll like it!

Ingredients

Taco cups

8-12 small purple cabbage leaves, as intact as possible

Taco "meat" filling

2 cups raw walnuts

1 Tbsp. cumin

1½ tsp. coriander

1½ tsp. onion powder

1 tsp. garlic powder, plus more, if desired

½ tsp. cayenne powder

Tamari

For assembly

Spring lettuce mix (or green leaves of your choice)

1 cup salsa; or make **Fresh Tomato Salsa** (see page 114)

1 cup guacamole; or make **Easy Guacamole** (see page 115)

Optional garnishes

Hot sauce, to taste

Sour cream; or make **Cashew Sour Cream** (see page 109)

Directions

Taco cups

Remove the outer leaves of a purple cabbage.

Try to remove the leaves one at a time, without breaking them. You want to make a "bowl" or taco shell out of each individual leaf. It may help you to cut off the bottom stem area to give greater access to the leaves. Soaking the cabbage in a bowl of cold water sometimes can also help to loosen up the leaves. When you have 8–12 leaves pulled off, set them aside.

Taco "meat" filling

Put all ingredients, except tamari, in a food processor and pulse until walnuts are finely chopped, but not oily. Add in the tamari little by little, a few tablespoons at a time, until the mixture begins to stick together. Taste as you go for the right balance of spices and tamari. When the mixture just starts to clump together it should be ready.

Assemble

Take one small leaf of the purple cabbage, place a small handful of mixed greens inside, followed by a large scoop of guacamole, and then sprinkle some taco meat on top. Add hot sauce and/or sour cream, if desired.

Beyond this recipe

This taco "meat" filling can be used in other uncooked recipes, as well. (Think Vegan Nachos or Salads.)

Did you know that walnuts have a higher antioxidant activity than any other common nut? Walnuts can help fight oxidative damage in your body, including damage due to LDL cholesterol. They are a great plant source of omega-3 fatty acids and help decrease inflammation in the body. Walnuts are a heart-healthy nut that also support strong brain function.

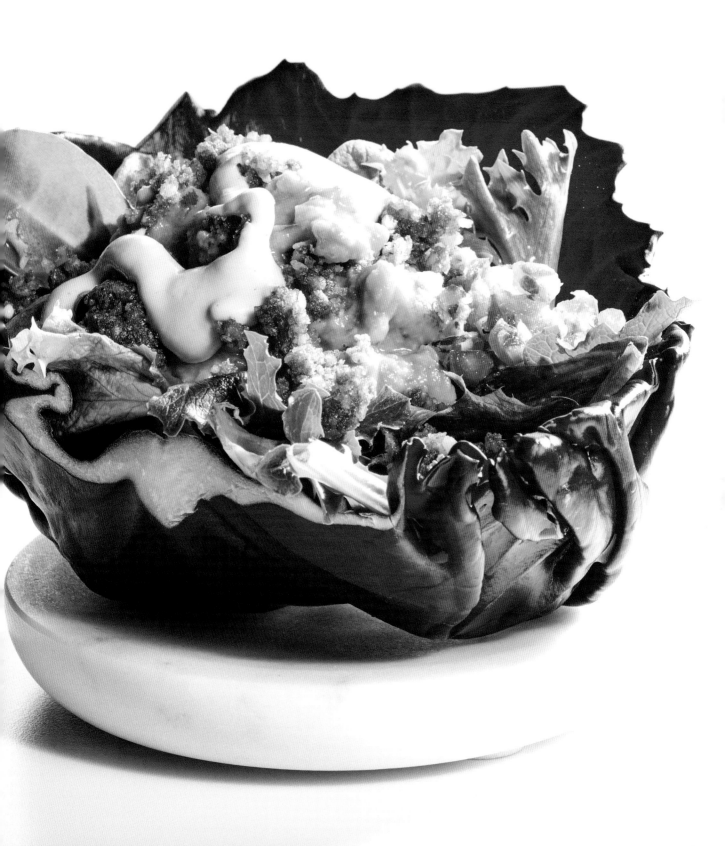

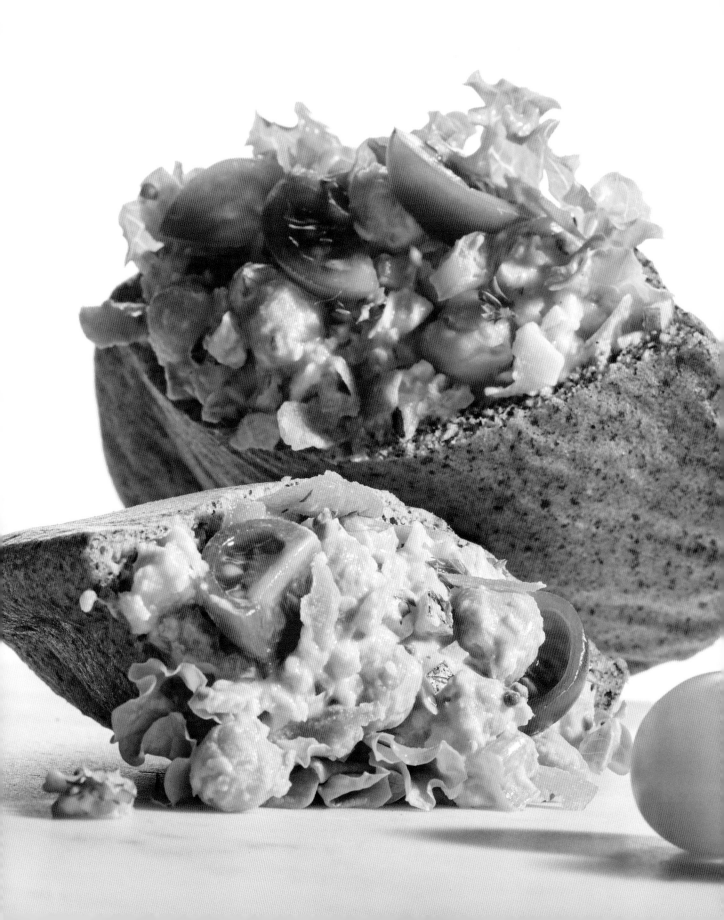

Yummy Chickpea Salad in a Pita Pocket

Makes 4 half-pita pockets.

This is a simple, but delicious, sandwich — it's a personal favorite.

Ingredients

Salad

- 1 15.5-oz. can chickpeas
- Water
- 1 medium stalk celery, finely diced
- ½ carrot, grated
- 1 Tbsp. red onion, finely minced
- 1 Tbsp. fresh parsley, chopped
- 3 Tbsp. mayonnaise or vegan mayonnaise
- 2 Tbsp. Dijon mustard
- 1–2 tsp. lemon juice
- ¼ tsp. salt

Sandwich

- 2 grain-free pita pockets or other grain-free bread; or make **Grain-free Pita Pockets** (see page 98)
- Lettuce, to taste
- Tomato, to taste

Directions

Salad

Rinse the chickpeas. Place in a saucepan covered with fresh water and heat until it just starts to boil. Remove from heat and drain liquid in a sieve. Transfer dry chickpeas to a bowl and mash with a fork until you achieve your preferred consistency. (A little chunky is nice.)

Add the remainder of the salad ingredients to the bowl and mix until uniformly combined. Adjust seasoning if desired.

Sandwich

Serve in a pita pocket with some lettuce and tomato.

Variation

You could also try this in a lettuce wrap, for a hand-held salad.

Serving suggestions

Try this for lunch in a pita pocket or serve it as a side dish for dinner with chicken or shrimp.

Chicken & Chickpea Chopped Salad with Creamy Cilantro Dressing

Makes 4 servings.

A salad that's a meal. Load up the ingredients — more is more!

Ingredients

Creamy cilantro dressing

1 cup loosely packed cilantro, stems removed and roughly chopped

½ cup plain Greek yogurt

¼ cup olive oil

2 Tbsp. fresh lime juice

1½ tsp. apple cider vinegar

1 soft medjool date, pit removed

1–2 garlic cloves

⅛ tsp. salt

Salad

1 lb. cooked, boneless skinless chicken breast, diced or shredded

Large head of romaine, chopped

1 15-oz. can chickpeas, rinsed and drained

1 large red or yellow bell pepper, seeds removed and diced

1 large or 2 small avocados, diced

1 pint cherry tomatoes, halved

4 green onions, chopped

Directions

Creamy cilantro dressing

Puree all ingredients in a blender or food processor until smooth. Taste and adjust seasonings, if necessary. Set aside.

Salad

Place all ingredients in a large bowl and mix with dressing to combine. You can also arrange toppings in sections with the dressing on the side for a beautiful visual effect.

Variation

Vegetarians can simply omit the chicken or add some hard-boiled egg or your favorite variety of bean for some extra protein.

Beyond this recipe

This creamy cilantro dressing could also be used as a topping for any salad, baked potatoes, or steamed vegetables.

Fresh cilantro is a rich source of many important vitamins, minerals, and therapeutic compounds, including vitamins A, C and K, calcium, potassium, magnesium, folate, and antioxidant flavonoids, phytonutrients, and phenols. It is an excellent source of fiber and contains virtually no calories.

Many people consider cilantro to be effective for individuals with diabetes. It can be good for digestive complaints. It can also help improve liver and heart function. Cilantro has the ability to bind harmful heavy metals in the body and loosen them from the tissues so that the body can eliminate them.

Cilantro works well in both cooked and raw recipes. Some people have a gene that makes cilantro taste like soap. If you are one of these people, feel free to substitute it with another fresh herb.

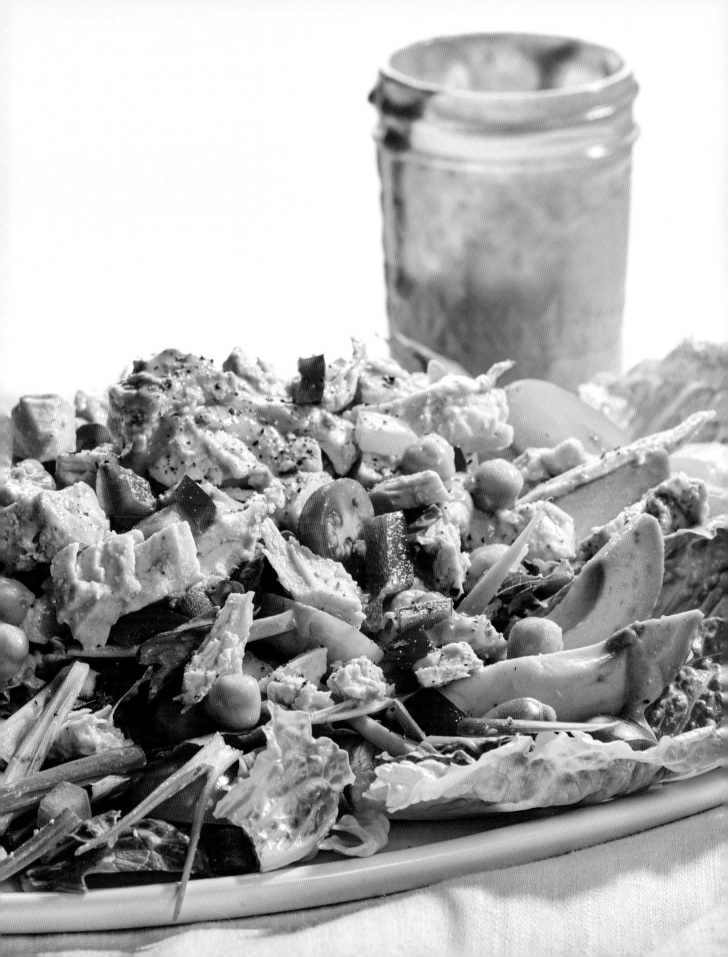

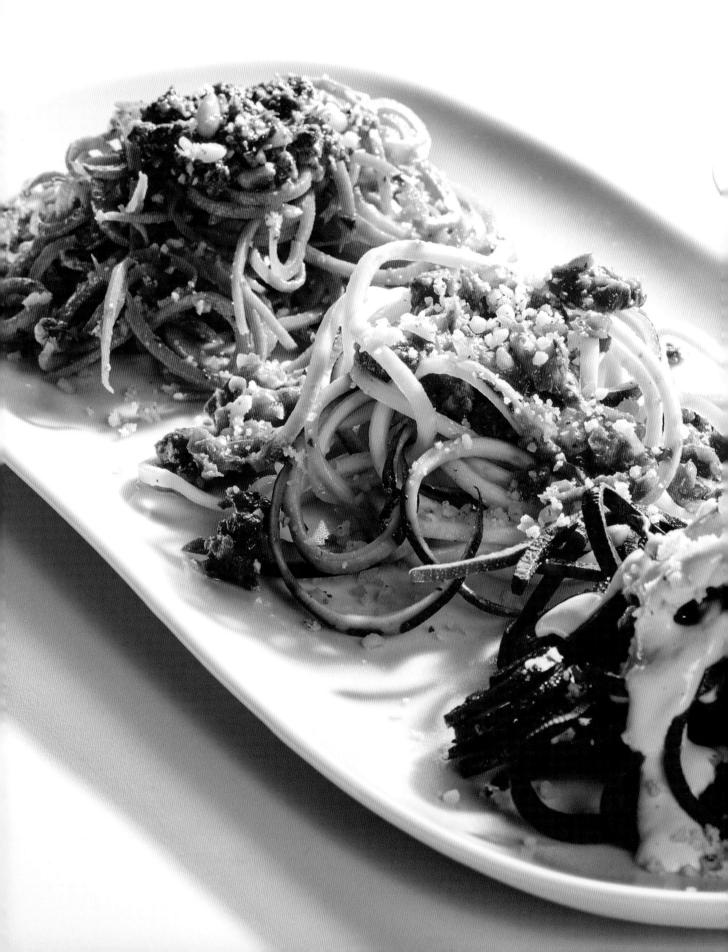

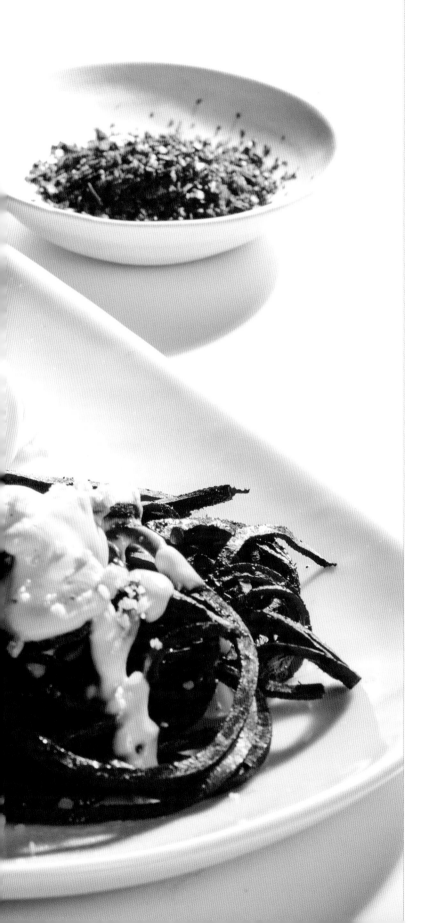

MAIN DISHES

Best-Ever Veggie Burger

Makes 4–6 burgers.

Tired of cardboard-tasting veggie burgers? I call these "Best-Ever" for good reason!

Ingredients

1 15-oz. can black beans, drained, rinsed, and patted dry

2 eggs (substitute with 3 Tbsp. ground flax, combined with hot water to form a paste, if vegan)

1 Tbsp. coconut oil or avocado oil

½ cup chickpea flour

½ cup mashed avocado

½ cup sundried tomatoes in olive oil, diced

½ cup feta cheese (optional)

½ medium red onion, finely diced

¼ cup fresh cilantro leaves, chopped (optional)

2 tsp. sweet or smoked paprika

1½ tsp. cumin

2 tsp. hot sauce (any kind)

2–3 small cloves of garlic, minced

1 tsp. salt

1 tsp. oregano

½ tsp. black pepper

Coconut or avocado oil

For assembly

4 low-carb burger buns; or make **(You Don't Need a Lettuce Wrap) Burger Buns** (see page 105)

Favorite burger condiments

Directions

Add black beans to a mixing bowl. Partially crush the beans with a fork, leaving some texture so the beans are not pulverized. Add the remaining ingredients, except the oil, and mix until the batter sticks together. (If using flax in place of the eggs, make sure the flax does not clump together. It should have a good consistency with the hot water, so that the batter holds together smoothly.)

Divide the burger mixture into 4–6 parts and mold each portion into a patty shape.

Heat some coconut or avocado oil in a frying pan on medium. Place the burgers into the hot pan and cook about 7 minutes on each side, turning occasionally.

Serve on a bun or lettuce wrap heaped with your favorite condiments.

Serving suggestions

Get creative with your condiments. Try sauerkraut, **Spicy Garlic Tomato Sauce** (see page 111), **Fresh Tomato Salsa** (see page 114), **Basil Pesto** (see page 74), **Easy Guacamole** (see page 115), or **Cashew Sour Cream** (see page 109).

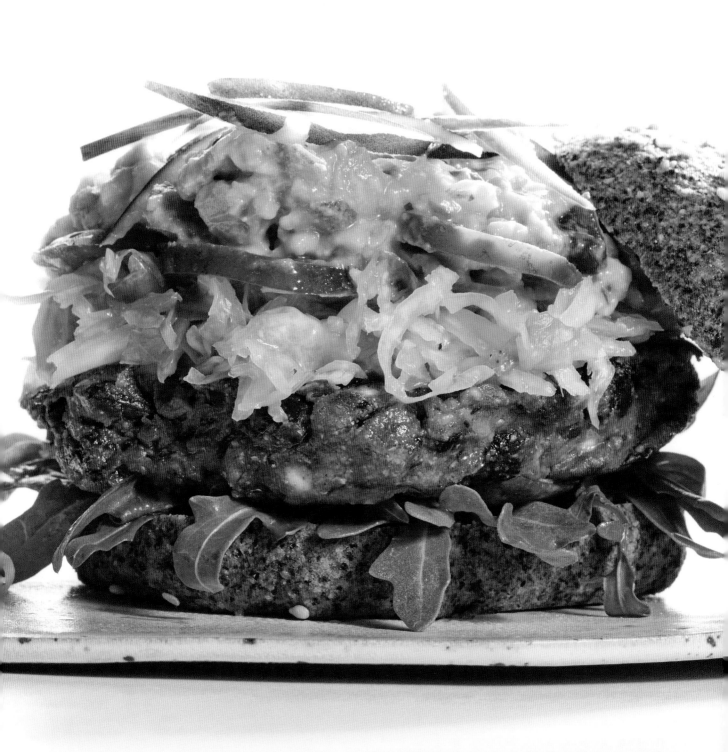

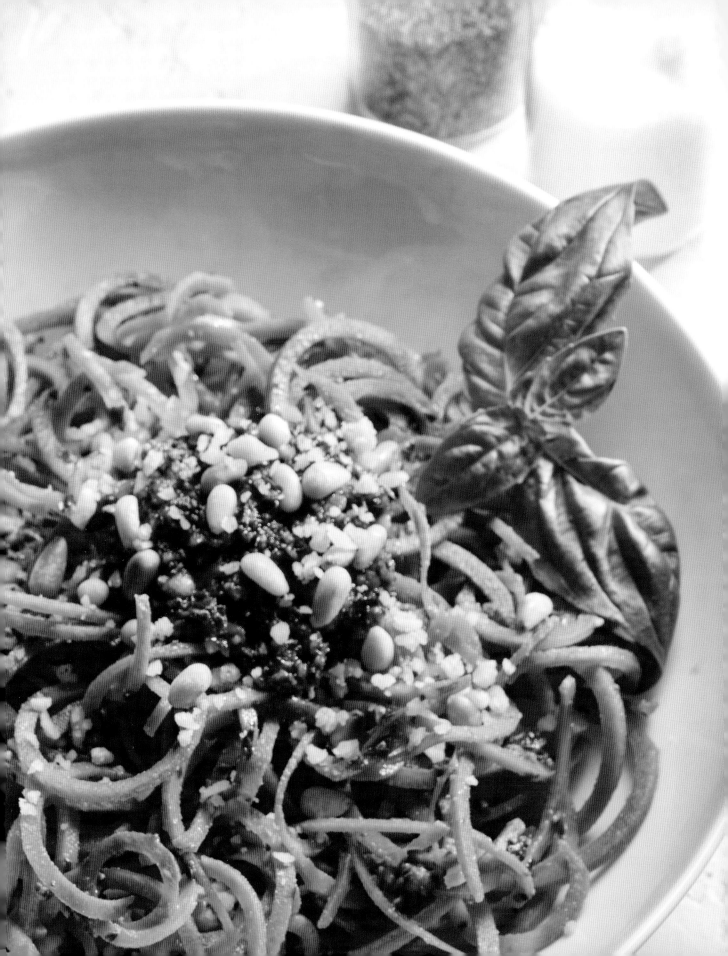

Colorful Vegetable Pasta

Make a beautiful display of different pasta noodles and sauces for a family meal, or simply choose one. Vegetable pasta lets you go to bed feeling light and able to sleep easily, since your body does not have to work so hard digesting all the heavy carbs of conventional pasta.

Noodles

Vegetable noodles are low in calories, low in carbohydrates, and aid in healthy digestion. They are gluten-free, so everyone can enjoy this pasta. They also have a high water content and are higher in fiber than traditional noodles. You get a lot more nutrition, without that bloated feeling. And vegetable noodles are quick and easy to make.

Most people use zucchini noodles as the base for vegetable pasta dishes, but you can also use carrot, beet, or squash noodles; kelp noodles; or shirataki noodles. All are low in sugars.

There are many spiralizer tools available to make noodles from a variety of vegetables. However, if you don't have a fancy machine, you can simply use a potato peeler to make strips of your vegetable—these noodles will resemble fettuccine.

Use your spiralizer (or peeler) to turn the zucchini/carrot/etc. into strips, ribbons, or noodles. Some people warm their noodles, but be careful not to overcook these, because they can become mushy (zucchini in particular). It's fine to keep the vegetable or kelp noodles raw and use the warm sauce with the acids to "cook" the noodles through marination. You will also get maximum nutrition this way. Alternatively—for tougher noodles like carrot and beet—heat them just 2 minutes in a sauté pan with a little butter, to soften them slightly. If you opt for shirataki noodles, you can sauté these for 2–3 minutes to warm.

Sauce

Once you have prepared your vegetable noodles, you can add any topping of your choice Basil Pesto Sauce, Creamy Faux Alfredo Sauce, or Marinara Sauce. The recipes for these are on the following pages.

Note

Make a large batch of your preferred sauce and freeze it in individual servings. That way, on a busy night, your meal is practically ready. Warm your sauces, spiralize your noodles, and you'll have dinner ready in 10 minutes, or less!

Serving suggestions

Top your noodles and sauce with capers, diced tomatoes, fresh basil, or parsley leaves, **Marinated Mushrooms** (see page 108), **Vegan Taco "Meat"** (see page 62), **Garlic Shrimp** (see page 82), and/or parmesan cheese. If you are dairy-free, try **Dairy-Free Parmesan Cheese** (see page 75).

Basil Pesto Sauce

Makes 6-8 servings.

I love homemade pesto. It's easy to make a big batch and freeze it in ice cube trays for convenient use in future recipes.

Ingredients

2 cups fresh basil leaves, tightly packed

3 Tbsp. olive oil

1 Tbsp. light miso paste

1 tsp. garlic, minced

1 tsp. nutritional yeast

½ tsp. salt

¼ cup pine nuts or walnuts

Directions

Combine all ingredients, except nuts, in a food processor. Using the "S" blade, pulse a few times to begin to chop the basil leaves.

Add the nuts and process until smooth. Be careful not to over-process the mixture, or the oil from the nuts will separate, and make the pesto feel greasy. The ideal texture should be creamy, with tiny specks of nuts throughout.

You can warm this sauce before serving or enjoy it at room temperature.

. . . .

Creamy Faux Alfredo Sauce

Makes 6-8 servings.

A surprising use of cashews! Rich, creamy, and delicious.

Ingredients

2 cups water

1½ cups raw cashews (unsalted)

2 Tbsp. avocado oil

½ medium sweet onion, chopped

4-5 cloves garlic, minced

2-3 Tbsp. fresh miso paste or ¼ cup nutritional yeast

1 Tbsp. lemon juice

1 tsp. salt, or to taste

Directions

Bring 2 cups of water to a boil. Pour the hot water over the cashews and let soak for 5 minutes. Set aside.

Heat the avocado oil in a sauté pan over medium heat. Once hot, add the onion and garlic and sauté for 5 minutes, until fragrant and the onion is translucent. Remove from heat.

Drain the cashews and discard the soaking water. Add the cashews and all the other ingredients, including onion and garlic, to a food processor, or high-performance blender. Blend until very smooth. Taste and adjust seasonings. Add additional water if the sauce is too thick. Add more soaked cashews if the sauce is too watery.

Serve warm.

Marinara Sauce

Makes 6–8 servings.

When making a sandwich, you can swap out your mayonnaise or mustard for this sauce (or either of the other two) as your spread. It can turn an ordinary lunch into something special.

Ingredients

2 regular or 3 Roma tomatoes, seeded and chopped

1 cup sun-dried tomatoes, packed in olive oil

½–1 red bell pepper, chopped

2 Tbsp. chopped red onion

½ cup fresh basil (or 2 tsp. dried basil)

¼ cup extra virgin olive oil

2 cloves garlic, crushed

1 Tbsp. pure maple syrup, not pancake syrup (optional)

1 Tbsp. lemon juice

1 tsp. dried oregano

½ tsp. salt, or to taste

Black pepper, to taste

Dash of cayenne pepper

Directions

Combine all ingredients in a food processor and pulse until well-combined, but still chunky.

You can warm the sauce lightly before serving or enjoy it at room temperature. This sauce does not require any further cooking.

Note

This sauce stores well in the fridge in a sealed glass jar.

Dairy-free Parmesan Cheese

Makes 6–8 servings.

This recipe for dairy-free Parmesan is fast, easy, and tastes great! It stores well in an airtight glass jar in the fridge or freezer and lasts for weeks.

Ingredients

1 cup Brazil nuts

1–2 cloves garlic

½ tsp. salt

Directions

Place all ingredients in a food processor and process until fine, but not oily. Sprinkle as desired, anywhere you would regularly use Parmesan cheese.

Keto Macro Bowl

Makes as many servings as needed, just follow the proportions.

This recipe allows for your creative juices to flow. Choose the ingredients you love most and keep to these proportions, using the quantities needed to satisfy your family or guests.

Ingredients

30% Greens
Start with a base of fresh mixed leafy greens: lettuce, spinach, steamed kale, arugula, or Swiss chard.

20% Low-carb grains
Add some quinoa or cauliflower rice, steamed (not more than ½ cup per serving).

30% Vegetables
Choose three to five raw vegetables: cucumber, diced tomato, sliced avocado, chopped zucchini, green beans, grated carrots, bell peppers, onion, beets, or roasted vegetables.

15% Protein
Pick one or two proteins: black beans, chickpeas, salmon, chicken, shrimp, tuna, boiled eggs, or **Veggie Burger** (see page 70).

5% Toppings
Top with a light amount of these: sauerkraut, seaweed, kimchi, pumpkin seeds, sprouts, hemp seeds, or microgreens.

Directions

Assemble all ingredients in a bowl. Strive for the balance noted above, so there will be plenty of color and texture.

Assemble
Finish your bowl with a couple of splashes of your favorite sauce or salad dressing.

Serving suggestions
Instead of using a store-bought sauce or salad dressing, try the **Tahini Dressing** (see page 114) or **Fresh Tomato Salsa** (see page 114).

Here's how to cook eggs to get that bright yellow, moist look and creamy mouth-feel texture. Add enough water in a pot to cover the eggs, and bring it to a low boil. Slowly lower each egg with a spoon into the boiling water so it doesn't crack. Continue to boil on low heat for 6 to 7 minutes, depending on how many eggs are in the pot. Remove eggs and allow to cool in cold water. Peel and enjoy.

Macro Bowls are a balanced way to get all the major macronutrients your body needs in one delicious meal. The variety of macro bowls is unlimited, but they traditionally contain brown rice.

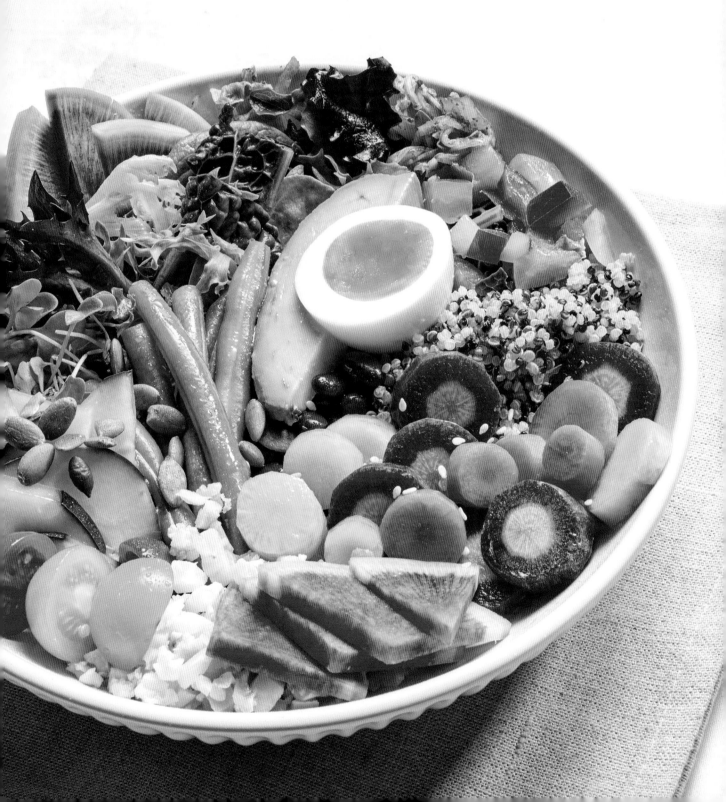

Black Bean & Avocado Sweet Potato Shells

Makes 4 servings.

Start off by oiling the potato skins to make them crispy and strong. Forget the foil or your potato shell will be too soft.

Ingredients

Potato shells

4 medium sweet potatoes
(roughly all the same size)

1–2 Tbsp. coconut oil or avocado oil

Salt, to taste, divided

Black pepper, to taste

For assembly

1 15-oz. can black beans (1½ cups cooked),
drained, rinsed and warmed

½ cup salsa; or make **Fresh Tomato Salsa**
(see page 114)

½ cup guacamole; or make **Easy Guacamole**
(see page 115)

Optional garnish

Sour cream; or make **Cashew Sour Cream**
(recipe page 109)

Directions

Preheat oven to 425°F. Line a baking tray with parchment paper.

Potato shells

Wash the sweet potatoes thoroughly and pat to dry. Poke holes in them with a fork or a knife to let the steam escape while cooking. Rub the outsides with some coconut or avocado oil. Season with a little salt/pepper on the oily skin.

Place the potatoes directly on the prepared tray. Bake for 45–60 minutes.

Assemble

At about 45 minutes, check the potatoes to see if they are done. Poke a fork into one potato. If it penetrates the potato easily, it is done. When fully baked, remove them from the oven. Slice each potato open, across the top, lengthwise, to allow the heat escape and keep the insides from getting too tough.

After the potatoes cool, scoop out 2/3 of the flesh from each potato and refrigerate for use elsewhere. You will now have 4 whole potato shells, with nice hollow openings and a still bit of baked potato lining inside.

Spoon about ¼ of the warm black beans into each shell and top that with a scoop each of the salsa and guacamole. Spoon on some sour cream, if you'd like. Serve immediately.

Beyond this recipe

Save the scooped out sweet potato flesh in a covered container. You can use it for **Egg Burrito** (see page 37). Or if you want a simple dish, you could whip it with butter, coconut cream, and salt to make a side of mashed sweet potatoes another day.

Salmon Fillets with Caramelized Onion

Makes 4 servings.

There is no substitute for the flavor of caramelized onions! This is a perfect dish for special occasions.

Ingredients

Caramelized onions

2 Tbsp. butter

2 yellow onions, julienned

Water, if needed

Salmon

4 fillets of salmon

Salt and black pepper, to taste

1 Tbsp. coconut oil or avocado oil

Sauce

3–4 cloves garlic, minced

½ pint mushrooms, sliced or 1 4-oz. can sliced mushrooms

¼ cup sundried tomatoes in oil, drained and diced

1 red or yellow bell pepper, julienned

1 Tbsp. coconut oil or avocado oil

¾ cup (6-oz. can) full fat coconut cream

¼ teaspoon smoked paprika

Salt and black pepper, to taste

Optional garnishes

1 small package of fresh, lightly wilted baby spinach leaves (see note)

2 Tbsp. capers

Juice from one lemon

Directions

Caramelized onions

In a medium skillet over medium heat, melt the butter. Add onion strips and cook, stirring often, until they start to soften. Reduce heat to medium-low and continue to stir, until the onions are soft, nicely brown, and sweet, 15–25 minutes. If the onions stick to the pan, add a little water to loosen.

When finished, put on a plate, and set aside.

Salmon

Season the salmon with salt and pepper.

Heat the oil in the same skillet you used for the onions, without cleaning it; this will add more flavor to the fish. Use medium-high heat. When the oil is hot, add the seasoned fillets of salmon, top side down. Sear for about 3–4 minutes, depending on thickness. Reduce heat to medium. Flip the salmon fillets to skin side down and sear another 3–4 minutes.

Remove from heat. Place on a plate and cover to keep warm.

Sauce

Add the garlic, mushrooms, sundried tomatoes, bell peppers, and caramelized onions to the same pan you prepared the fish in. Stir in a little more oil, and cook over medium-high heat until tender. Add the coconut cream and paprika and mix, until combined and evenly heated. Season with salt and pepper.

Assemble

Add the salmon back into the skillet with the sauce to warm through. Remove from heat and serve on a bed of lightly wilted spinach. Serve the fish and spinach topped with capers and a squeeze of fresh lemon.

Note

To wilt spinach, wash and drain it, but do not pat dry. Toss the damp leaves in a dry pan and lightly heat, until it has softened.

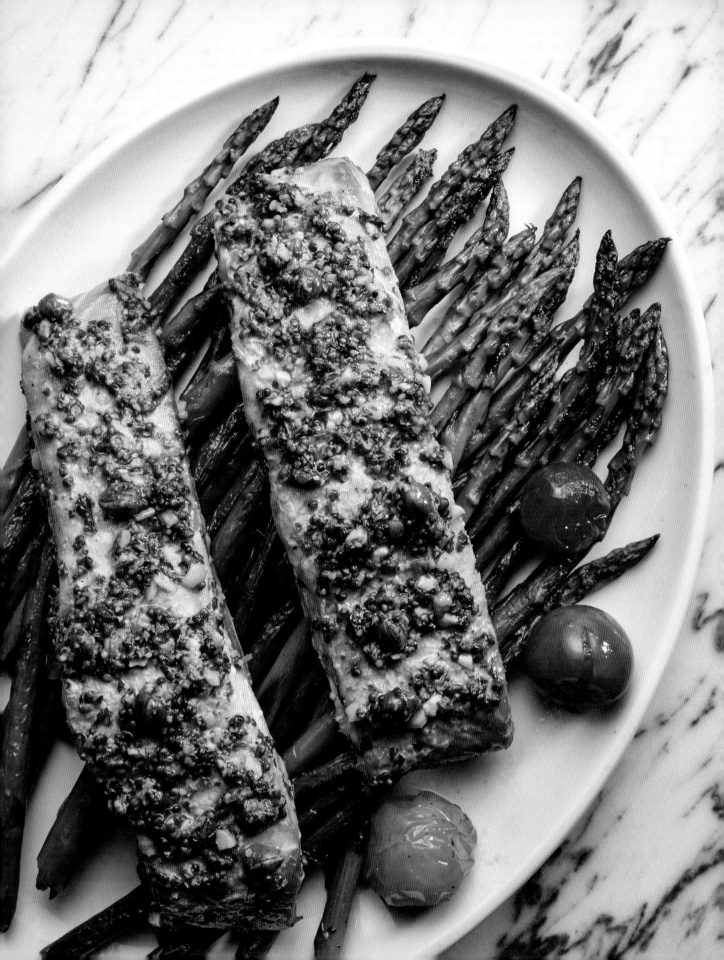

Dijon Salmon with Capers

Makes 4 servings.

When you're in the mood for a fancy meal.

Ingredients

2 Tbsp. butter, at room temperature

¼ cup Dijon mustard

¼ cup fresh parsley, finely chopped

3–4 cloves garlic, minced

2–3 Tbsp. capers

Salt and black pepper, to taste

1½ lbs. salmon, preferably wild-caught

Optional garnishes

Juice of 1 lemon

Splash of olive oil or extra melted butter

Directions

Preheat oven to 375°F. Line a baking tray with parchment paper.

Mix the butter, mustard, parsley, garlic, capers, salt, and pepper in a small bowl.

Place the salmon, skin side down, on the tray. Coat the top of the salmon generously with the herbed mustard mix.

Bake for 18–20 minutes, depending on size and thickness. When salmon is finished (cooked through and flaky), remove from oven and slice into individual portions. Do not overcook, since the salmon will continue to cook, even after you remove it from the oven.

Squeeze a bit of lemon juice with a dash of olive oil on top of each portion before serving.

Serving suggestions

This meal would pair well with some **Garlic Greens** (see page 106), **Kale Salad with Pistachios & Cranberries** (see page 58), or **Kelp Noodle Salad** (see page 56).

Garlic Shrimp with Cauliflower Veggie Fried Rice

Makes 4 servings.

I love garlic and when everyone at the table indulges — then there are no worries about garlicky breath!

Ingredients

Garlic shrimp

20 large or jumbo shrimp, raw, peeled, and deveined

2 Tbsp. chopped garlic

¾ cup fresh parsley

2 tsp. paprika

Salt and black pepper, to taste

⅓ cup avocado oil

2 Tbsp. butter

Cauliflower veggie fried rice

1 head cauliflower

2 Tbsp. coconut oil or avocado oil

½ cup fresh spinach, finely chopped

¼ cup red or yellow bell pepper, finely chopped

¼ cup carrot, finely chopped

¼ cup onion, finely diced

1 tsp. ginger, finely grated

3 cloves fresh garlic, finely minced

1 green chili, finely minced

Swish of toasted sesame oil

1 Tbsp. tamari

1 tsp. rice vinegar (or substitute apple cider vinegar)

¼ tsp., plus a pinch salt, divided

¼ tsp. black pepper

2 eggs

Optional garnishes

Small handful fresh cilantro leaves

Green onion

Sriracha, to taste

Directions

Garlic shrimp

Mix all the shrimp ingredients together in a large bowl and cover tightly with plastic wrap or aluminum foil. Refrigerate and allow to marinate for at least an hour. While the shrimp marinate, prepare the rice.

Cauliflower veggie fried rice

Chop cauliflower into small chunks. Then use a food processor to grate the cauliflower into smaller, rice-sized pieces. Or you can do this by hand with a knife or grater.

In a non-stick sauté pan, heat the avocado or coconut oil. Add the cauliflower, all the finely chopped vegetables, ginger, garlic, and chili. Heat on high for 5–6 minutes.

Add the seasonings, including sesame oil (add sparingly), tamari, vinegar, salt, and pepper. Stir to combine.

Crack eggs in a small bowl. Add a pinch of salt and whisk. Make a well in the pan, in the middle of the vegetables, and add the egg. Stir gently until almost scrambled. Mix the contents of the pan with the egg.

Garnish with cilantro leaves and/or chopped green onion. Add a splash of sriracha if you'd like.

Assemble

After the shrimp have marinated, melt the butter in a large saucepan on medium heat. Add the shrimp and toss around for approximately 8–10 minutes, until pink and lightly browned. Do not overcook, or else the shrimp will get rubbery. Serve immediately, while warm, on top of the Fried Cauliflower Veggie Rice.

Serving suggestion

The Garlic Shrimp, without the rice, would make a nice topper for the **Vegetable Pasta** (see page 73) with **Marinara Sauce** (see page 75).

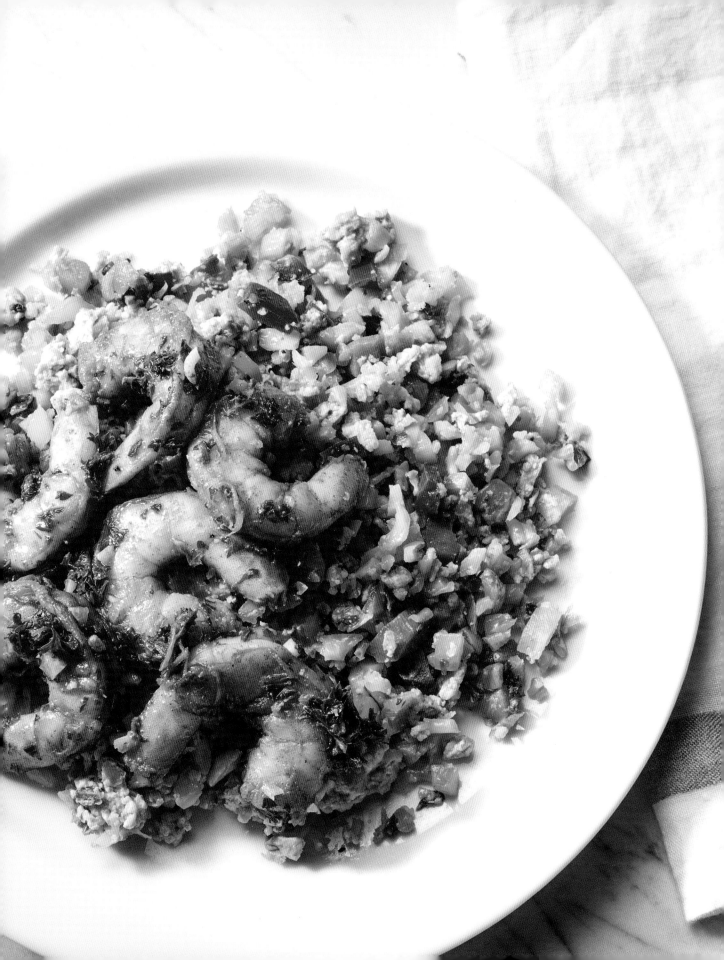

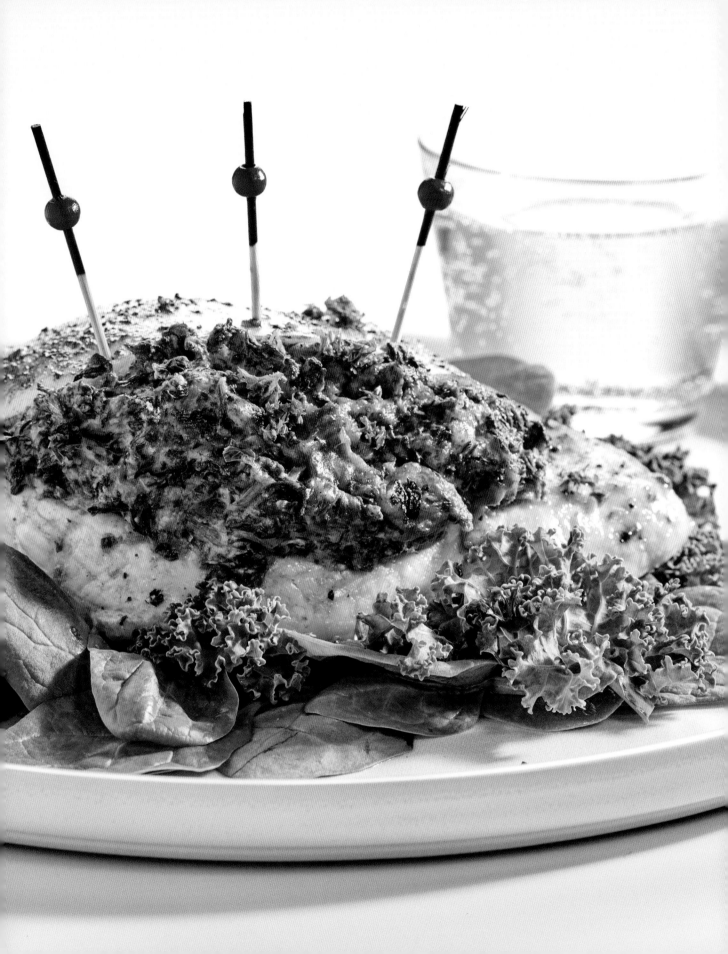

Spinach-Stuffed Chicken Breast

Makes 4 servings.

Easy and delicious — what better way to eat your greens?

Ingredients

4 cups fresh spinach (or 1 10-oz. pkg frozen), chopped

4 oz. cream cheese, at room temperature

¼ cup grated Parmesan cheese

¼ cup mozzarella cheese

1 tsp. fresh garlic, minced

1 tsp. smoked paprika

½ tsp. chili powder

1 tsp. salt, divided

½ tsp. black pepper, divided

4 chicken breasts, bone removed, skin optional

¼ tsp. garlic powder

1 Tbsp. coconut oil or avocado oil, or butter, melted

Directions

Preheat oven to 375°F.

If you are using frozen spinach, thaw it and squeeze it to remove as much moisture as possible.

In a non-stick sauté pan, add the soft cream cheese and chopped spinach. Stir until well mixed and spinach is wilted. Add the Parmesan, mozzarella, minced garlic, paprika, chili, and half of the salt and pepper.

Cut a large pocket, at an angle, into your raw chicken breasts, being careful not to slice all the way through. Season the chicken breast with garlic powder, and remaining salt and pepper. Fill each of the pockets with ¼ of the spinach mixture, then close and seal with toothpicks.

Place the stuffed chicken into a baking dish and drizzle with oil or melted butter. Bake approximately 25–30 minutes, until chicken is cooked through.

When chicken is fully cooked, remove from oven and let rest, covered, for a few minutes. Pull out the toothpicks before serving.

Variation

Substitute steamed broccoli for the spinach.

Serving suggestions

Try this with **Cauliflower Rice** (see page 108) or **Marinated Mushrooms** (see page 108).

Mushroom Artichoke Pesto Chicken

Makes 4 servings.

Serve this to your family or at your next dinner party to impress the guests — it's scrumptious!

Ingredients

Chicken

2 large or 4 small boneless skinless chicken breasts (1–1½ lbs.)

1 Tbsp. coconut or avocado oil, plus more, if needed

Mushroom artichoke pesto sauce

3–4 cloves garlic, minced

1 pint cherry tomatoes, halved

1 pint mushrooms, sliced

1 medium zucchini, cut into chunks

1 cup marinated artichoke pieces, drained

¼ cup basil pesto; or make **Basil Pesto Sauce** (see rpage 74)

½ cup full-fat coconut cream

1 teaspoon paprika

¼ teaspoon chili powder

Salt and black pepper, to taste

Directions

Chicken

If you have 2 large chicken breasts, slice them evenly horizontally to make 4 thinner pieces; one for each serving.

In a large, warm skillet, add the oil, then the chicken. Cook the chicken on medium high heat for 3–4 minutes on each side or until no longer pink in the center. Remove chicken and set aside on a plate.

Mushroom artichoke pesto sauce

Add a little more oil to the same pan, if needed. Toss in garlic, tomatoes, mushrooms, zucchini, and artichokes. Cook over medium-high heat, until tender. Add the pesto and coconut cream. Stir together, until well-combined and evenly cooked. Add the spices and season with salt and pepper.

Assemble

Put the chicken back into the skillet with the sauce to warm through. Serve immediately.

Serving suggestions

This chicken is tasty with some steamed broccoli, or **Garlic Greens** (see page 106) on the side, or on top of a bed of **Kelp Noodle Salad** (see page 56).

Chicken Caesar Quesadillas with Bacon

Makes 4 quesadillas.

Looking for a game-time diabetic-friendly snack or a light meal? This one is easy and appealing!

Ingredients

Butter or coconut or avocado oil, or cooking spray, divided

1 small red onion, diced

4 low-carb tortillas or wraps; or make **Herbed Tortilla Wraps** (see page 100)

2 cups shredded rotisserie chicken (or leftover turkey)

8 slices cooked bacon (any kind), chopped or broken into bite-sized pieces

$\frac{1}{3}$ cup Caesar dressing

1 $\frac{1}{3}$ cup shredded cheddar cheese

Optional garnishes

Salsa; or make **Fresh Tomato Salsa** (see page 114), to taste

Guacamole; or make **Easy Guacamole** (see page 115), to taste

Directions

Preheat oven to 300°F.

Heat a little butter, oil, or cooking spray in a sauté pan. When warm, toss in the diced onion and sauté a few minutes to soften. Set aside on a plate.

Heat the pan again with a little more butter, or oil, then add one of the tortillas to the pan on a low, medium heat.

On top of half the tortilla, add your chopped or shredded chicken or turkey, 2–3 Tbsp. bacon pieces (about 2 slices), a sprinkle of the sautéed onions and 1$\frac{1}{2}$ Tbsp. of Caesar dressing. On the other half of the tortilla, add about $\frac{1}{3}$ cup shredded cheese. Allow the cheese to melt, being careful not to burn the tortilla; about 4–5 minutes.

Once the cheese has melted, flip half of the tortilla onto the other half, so it is folded into a half-moon shape.

Remove from pan and place on a baking tray in the warmed oven. Repeat the process with the remaining tortillas, until all are finished.

To serve, cut each folded tortilla into thirds and serve with a dollop of guacamole and a spoonful of salsa.

Variation

Switch out the Caesar dressing for your favorite dressing or sauce.

Curried Chicken Skillet

Makes 4 servings.

A full meal prepared in one pan. Easy prep and easy cleanup, too!

Ingredients

2-3 Tbsp. coconut oil or avocado oil

1 lb. boneless skinless chicken breast, cut into bite-sized pieces

1 medium/large onion, diced

3 cloves garlic, finely minced

2-3 tsp. ground ginger or 1 Tbsp. fresh ginger, finely minced

2 tsp. coriander

3 medium carrots, grated

¼ cup sundried tomatoes in olive oil, diced

1 13-oz. can coconut milk or ½ cup coconut cream, plus ½ cup water

2 Tbsp. curry powder

1 tsp. salt, or to taste

½ tsp. black pepper, or to taste

3 cups fresh spinach leaves, chopped

1 Tbsp. lime juice

Dash of hot sauce

Optional garnish

¼ cup fresh cilantro, finely chopped

Directions

Put the oil, chicken, and onion into a large skillet. Sauté over medium-high heat, until the onion begins to soften, and the chicken is no longer pink—about 5 minutes. Stir occasionally.

Add the garlic, ginger, coriander, carrots, and sundried tomatoes. Cook for about 1 minute, stirring frequently.

Add the coconut milk or cream/water, curry powder, salt, and pepper. Stir to combine. Reduce the heat to medium, and allow mixture to simmer for about 5 minutes, or until liquid volume has reduced and the mixture has thickened slightly.

Add the chopped spinach, lime juice, and hot sauce, and stir to combine. Cook until spinach has wilted and is tender, about 1 to 2 minutes. Taste and adjust seasoning as desired.

Garnish with cilantro and serve immediately.

Note

You can use shredded rotisserie chicken to save time.

Variation

To make this a vegetarian dish, use one 15-oz. can chickpeas, rinsed and drained, instead of chicken.

Serving suggestion

This pairs well with **Cheezy Broccoli** (see page 107).

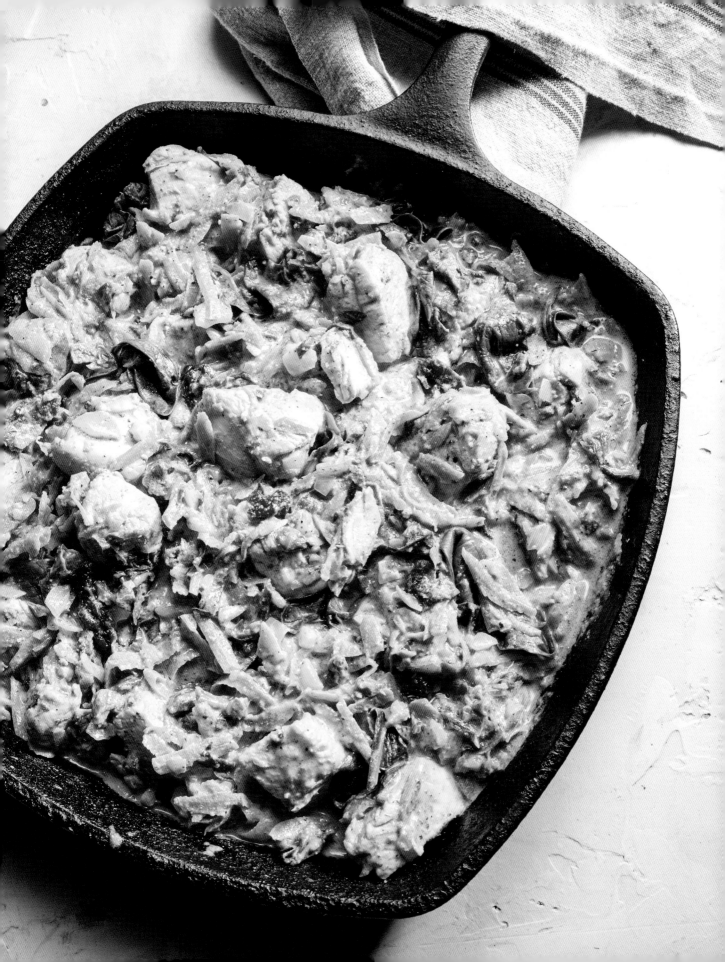

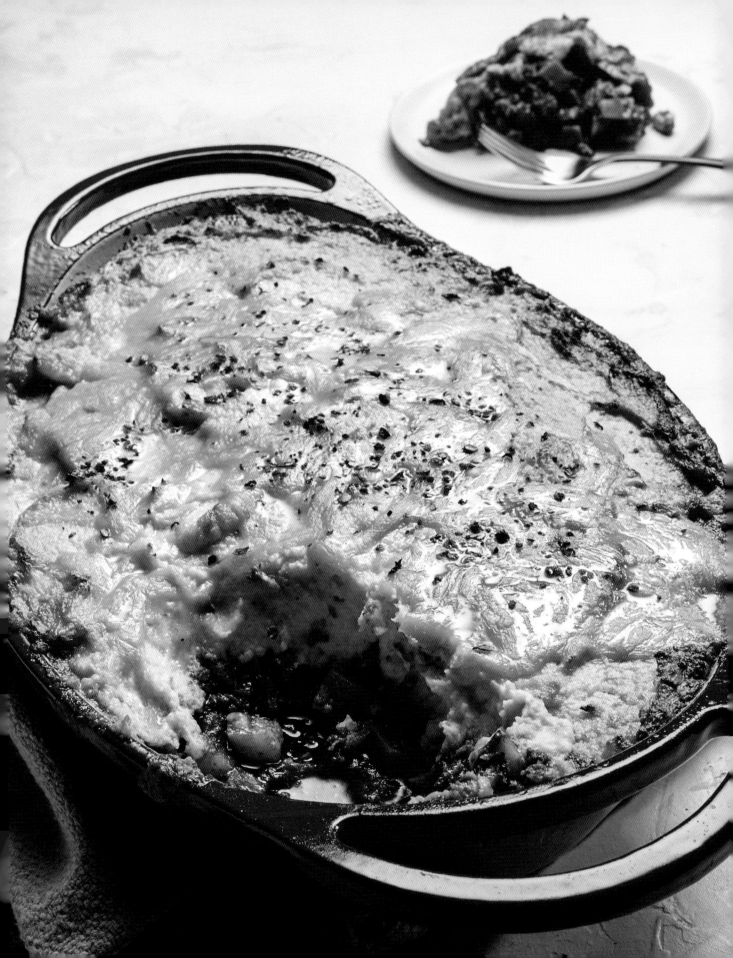

Low-Carb Shepherd's Pie

Makes 4–6 servings.

Whether you call this Shepherd's Pie or Cottage Pie, what is special about this dish is the creamy cauliflower topping. (You won't miss the mashed potatoes usually used.) This pie is spot-on for comfort food!

Ingredients

Base

    1 Tbsp. avocado or coconut oil
    1 small onion, diced
    6 cloves garlic, minced
    1 lb. ground beef (or bison)
    3 stalks celery, finely chopped
    1 small zucchini, diced
    2 carrots, finely chopped
    ½ cup mushrooms, finely chopped
    1 28-oz. can crushed tomatoes
    1 Tbsp. parsley flakes
    1 Tbsp. fresh thyme, finely minced
    1 Tbsp. fresh rosemary, finely minced
    Salt and black pepper, to taste

Topping

    1 head cauliflower, cut into florets
    Water
    2 Tbsp. butter
    ½ cup coconut cream or 3 oz. cream cheese
    ½ tsp. onion powder
    Salt and black pepper, to taste

Optional

    1 cup cheddar cheese, freshly grated
    Paprika and/or chili powder, to taste

Directions

Preheat oven to 350°F. Generously butter or oil a large casserole dish.

Base

Heat oil in a large sauté pan.

Add the onion and garlic and cook a few minutes on medium heat until soft and translucent. Add the ground beef and cook through, stirring frequently, until browned. Add the celery, zucchini, carrot, mushrooms, tomatoes, and spices. Stir to combine.

Reduce the heat to a simmer and continue cooking on low, uncovered for 10 minutes, or until most of the liquid evaporates.

Topping

In a steamer (or large pot with a small amount of water), steam the cauliflower until soft, about 8–10 minutes. Drain the water, then allow the cauliflower to cool slightly.

Transfer the dry cauliflower to a blender or food processor. Add the butter, cream or cream cheese, onion powder, salt, and pepper, and process until smooth. Set aside.

Assemble

Place the ground beef mixture in the prepared casserole dish. Spread the mashed cauliflower mixture on top and sprinkle with grated cheese. Dust with a pinch of paprika or chili powder for color, if desired.

Bake 25–30 minutes, until the filling is bubbly and the topping has browned.

Variation

Try this recipe with your favorite vegan or vegetarian ground beef substitute.

Crustless Taco Pie

Makes 8 servings.

An easy family meal, especially if you prepare the seasoning mix in advance.

Ingredients

Taco seasoning

2 Tbsp. chili powder

2 tsp. salt

2 tsp. cumin powder

2 tsp. garlic powder

1½ tsp. smoked paprika

1 tsp. black pepper

½ tsp. dried oregano

½ tsp. onion powder

⅛ tsp. cayenne pepper , to taste

Taco pie

1 lb. ground beef (or bison)

Dash of avocado or coconut oil, if needed

3 Tbsp. taco seasoning (recipe above)

⅔ cup coconut cream

4 large eggs

⅛ cup chunky salsa

1¼ cup sharp cheddar cheese, freshly grated, divided

2 cloves garlic, minced

½ tsp. salt

¼ tsp. black pepper

Splash of hot sauce (optional)

Optional garnishes

Guacamole; or make **Easy Guacamole** (see page 115)

Sour cream; or make **Cashew Sour Cream** (see page 109)

Salsa; or make **Fresh Tomato Salsa** (see page 114)

Cilantro leaves, chopped

Pickled jalapeños, chopped

Directions

Preheat an oven to 350°F. Grease a 9" pie pan and set aside.

Taco seasoning

Stir all ingredients together. Store extra seasoning in an airtight glass jar for use in other recipes that call for a little kick of spice.

Taco pie

Brown the ground beef in a sauté pan, adding oil, if needed, to keep the beef from sticking. Drain any grease. Add the taco seasoning to the ground beef in the same pan and stir it to combine. Put the seasoned taco beef into the greased pie pan.

In a small bowl, combine the coconut cream and eggs. Add the salsa, ¾ cup of the shredded cheese, garlic, salt, pepper, and hot sauce. Stir, then pour the egg mixture over the taco beef in the pie pan. Top the pie evenly with the rest of the shredded cheese.

Bake uncovered for 35 to 40 minutes, or until the center is set and the top is golden brown. Let cool 5 minutes before serving.

Top with your favorite garnishes, like those suggested here.

Note

Pre-shredded packets of cheese contain potato starch. It is used to prevent the cheese from sticking together. Grate your own cheese to avoid these extra carbs.

Variation

To make a lighter version of this recipe, you can use ground turkey or chicken instead of beef and reduce the amount of cheese.

Caramelized Onion & Mushroom Beef Burger Sliders

Makes 8 small burgers.

Make these into small burgers, like sliders, or larger ones for a full-sized appetite.

Ingredients

4 oz. can mushrooms, chopped; or ½ cup fresh, diced; or ½ cup **Marinated Mushrooms** (see page 108)

1 small onion (red or yellow), finely diced

1–2 tsp. butter

1½–2 tsp. minced garlic

24 oz. grass-fed ground beef (or bison)

1 egg

3 Tbsp. almond flour

1 Tbsp. Worcestershire sauce

1 tsp. chili powder

1 tsp. paprika

½ tsp. salt

¼ tsp. black pepper

For assembly

8 small low-carb burger buns; or make **(You Don't Need a Lettuce Wrap) Burger Buns** (see page 105), toasted

Favorite burger condiments

Directions

Dice the mushrooms and onion into similar size pieces. If using fresh mushrooms, the marinated version is tasty, but not necessary.

Sauté the diced onion with a little butter in a pan on medium low heat slowly until caramelized, stirring occasionally to prevent burning. When the onions are nearly browned, add the diced mushroom and minced garlic. Stir until well combined. Let cool.

In a mixing bowl, add the onion/mushroom mixture and all the other ingredients. Stir together until all ingredients are evenly distributed. Be careful not to overmix or the meat will become tough. With lightly damp hands (to prevent sticking), form the beef into eight 3-oz. patties.

Place the burgers in the refrigerator. You will want to start cooking the burgers when they are still cold—not at room temperature—to maximize flavor and juiciness. (While the patties are chilling, you can prepare the rest of your meal.)

Once the burgers are cold, place them in a large, warm skillet or grill. No need to add oil. Cook about 3–4 minutes each side, or until you reach the desired temperature (125°–145° F depending on how well-done you like your burgers). Resist the urge to flip the burgers more than once. Do not press down on them while cooking; this will squeeze out the internal juices and dry them out.

Remove the burgers from the grill or skillet and let them rest a few minutes. Serve on a toasted bun with your favorite condiments.

Variations

For a modern twist, serve your burgers in an **Herbed Tortilla Wrap** (see page 100). You could also try a lettuce leaf wrap, instead of a bun.

Crispy Carnitas on Jicama Wraps

Makes 4 servings.

The jicama wrap makes this a great variation on a Mexican classic.

Ingredients

Carnitas

2 lbs. pork shoulder, cut into large chunks

2 tsp. salt, divided

1 Tbsp. avocado or coconut oil

¾ cup chicken broth

¼ cup orange juice

Juice of 2 limes

1 medium onion, diced

4 cloves garlic, minced

1 tsp. paprika

1 tsp. dried oregano

1 tsp. dried parsley

1 tsp. cumin powder

½ tsp. black pepper

Red pepper flakes (optional)

Wraps

1 fresh jicama, or pre-made wraps

Optional garnishes

Shredded lettuce, to taste

Pickled red onion, to taste

Black beans, to taste

Guacamole, to taste

Fresh cilantro, to taste

Lime wedges, to taste

Salsa of choice, to taste

Directions

Preheat oven to 300°F.

Carnitas

Heat a large oven-proof sauté pan over medium-high heat. While the pan is warming, sprinkle the pork pieces liberally with salt. Once the pan is hot, add a tablespoon of oil and then add the pork. Sear for 4–5 minutes on each side, until browned.

Add the chicken broth, orange juice, lime juice, onion, garlic, salt, and the rest of the carnitas spices to the pan. Stir until combined, then cover with a lid. Braise in the oven for 3 hours or cook on high in a slow cooker for 4–6 hours, until the meat is fork-tender.

Once the pork is tender, remove it from the oven (or slow cooker) and transfer it to a rimmed sheet pan. Use two forks to shred the meat. Then pour the remaining braising liquid (up to a cup) back over the meat. Turn your oven to Broil and cook the carnitas until the edges begin to brown and get crispy, about 10–15 minutes.

Wraps

If using a fresh jicama, start with it whole. Peel the jicama to remove the outer skin. Using a mandoline, or sharp knife, cut the jicama into thin (no thicker than ¹/₈") round slices.

Assemble

Use your jicama slices like small tortilla wraps. Place some crispy carnitas in each wrap, along with your favorite garnishes, like those suggested and fold them in half, like a taco.

Variation

You can often find a tasty jackfruit pork substitute for vegetarians and those who want to avoid pork.

Jicama wraps are a gluten-free alternative to traditional wraps made with grains. Jicama is refreshing and has crunchy texture with a mild sweet flavor, so it's a perfect alternative for healthier dishes.

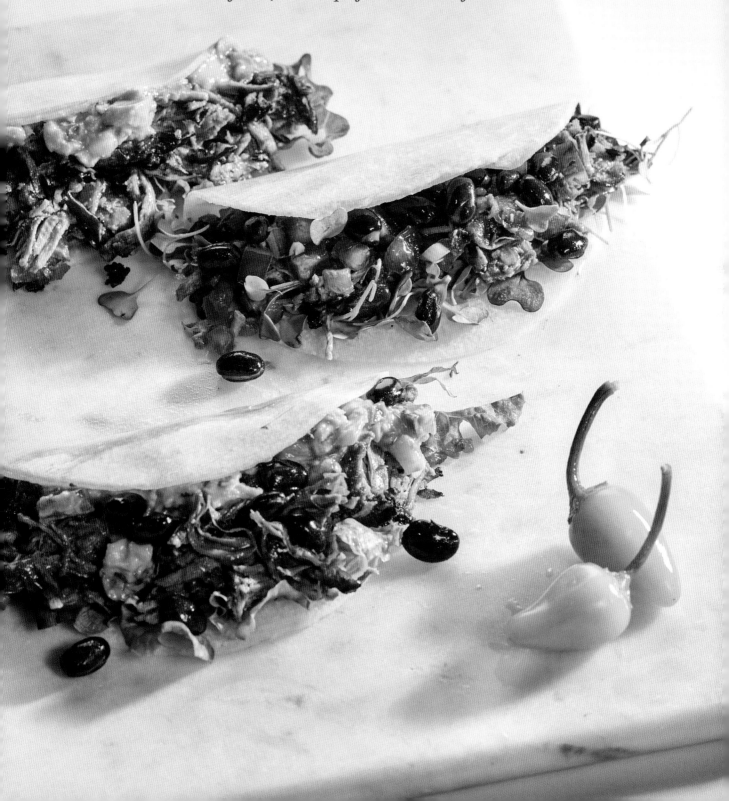

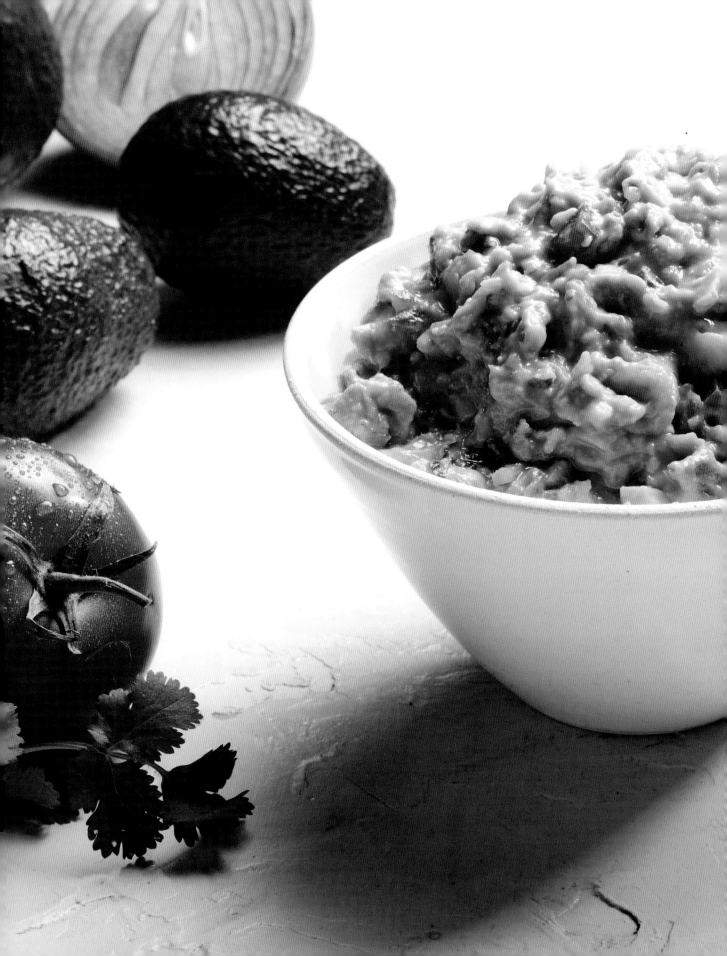

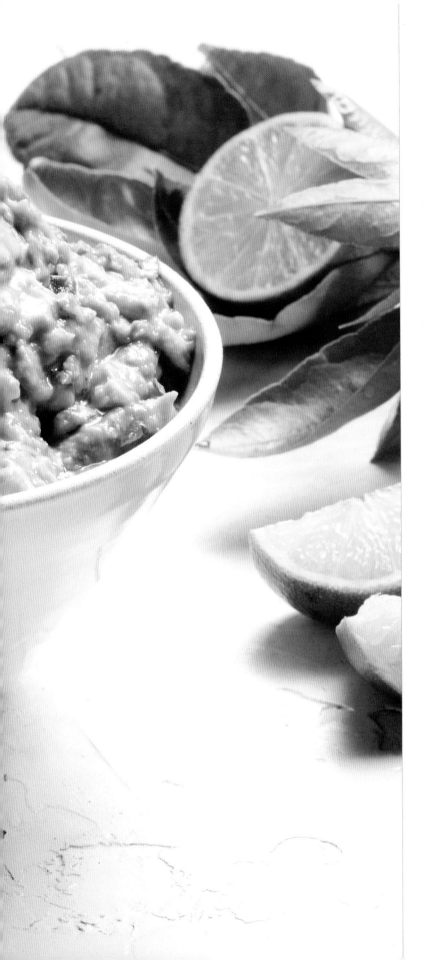

BREADS, SIDES & CONDIMENTS

Grain-Free Pita Pockets

Makes 4 pita pockets.

You will get so much satisfaction knowing you made your own bread — and they taste great, too!

Ingredients

½ cup hot water

2 eggs

½ cup almond flour, firmly packed

2 Tbsp. chickpea flour

2 tsp. psyllium husk powder
(for pliability)

1–2 tsp. za'atar spice blend

¼ tsp. baking soda

¼ tsp. salt

Directions

Preheat oven to 350°F. Line a baking tray with parchment paper.

Add water and eggs to a medium mixing bowl and whisk to combine. Add in dry ingredients and whisk. This will form a thick batter.

Evenly divide the batter into 4 circles about ½" high onto the baking tray.

Bake in the oven 18–20 minutes. Remove from the heat and let cool on a wire rack. Cut each circle in half. Then, using a good, sharp knife, carefully slice a slit in each pita half to make a pocket. Fill with the ingredients of your choice.

Note

This is best served fresh or store in an airtight container in the refrigerator for up to a couple of days.

Variations

Use different spices to change the flavor of the pitas. Try an Italian blend to go with your zucchini noodles and marinara dinner, add nutritional yeast to make a slightly cheesy flavor, or use cinnamon for a slightly sweet treat.

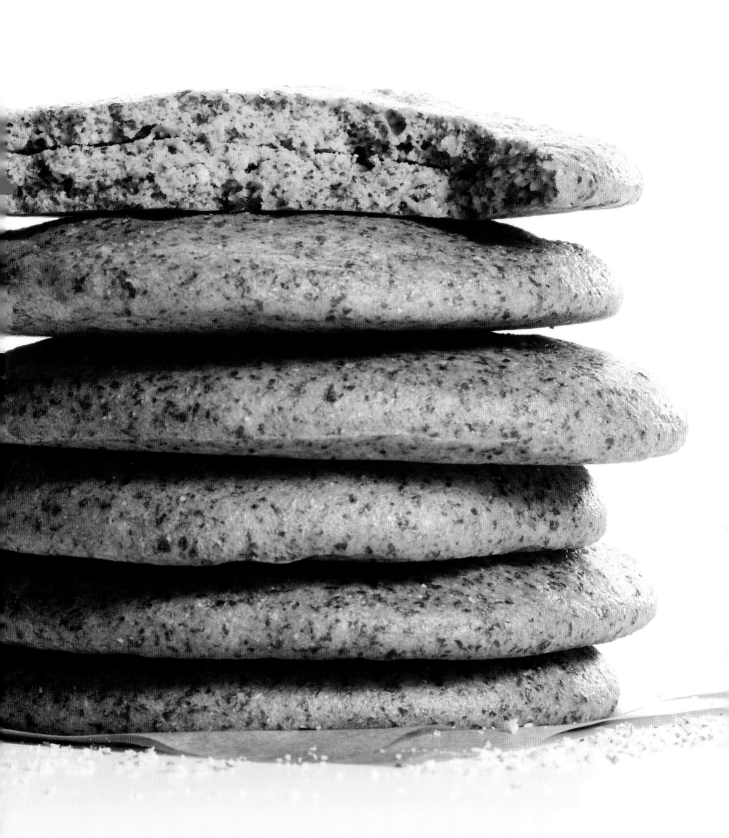

Herbed Tortilla Wraps

Makes 2–3 wraps.

Make these in advance and pull them out of the fridge in a pinch for easy meals or snacks.

Ingredients

- ¼ cup almond flour
- 2 Tbsp. chickpea flour
- 2 tsp. psyllium husk powder
- 2 tsp. flax seeds, freshly ground into a meal via a coffee grinder
- 1 tsp. sundried tomato powder
- ½ tsp. garlic powder
- ¼ tsp. baking soda
- ¼ tsp. salt
- 1 Tbsp. coconut oil, melted
- 1 Tbsp. egg white (about half of 1 egg)
- ⅓ cup boiling water

Directions

Mix all dry ingredients together in a bowl. Incorporate well.

Add the coconut oil and egg white to the dry ingredients and mix with a fork. Pour boiling water in, stirring quickly to incorporate. The dough will absorb the water and become easy to work with. Depending on how thick the consistency of the dough is, you may need to add more water. Strive for a consistency that sticks together, but is pliable.

Divide the dough in half or thirds. Roll each portion into a ball, then place in between two parchment sheets. Flatten out to about ¼" high.

Place flattened dough in a pre-heated dry non-stick skillet or tortilla press. Cook 2–3 minutes, pressing the dough with a spatula and flipping to cook both sides, if using a skillet.

Note

Psyllium powder is usually available at your local health food store or easily obtainable online. It really helps keep these tortillas soft and pliable.

Variations

Substitute other spice blends instead of the ones suggested here, as desired. Try Italian herbs, turmeric, za'atar, etc.

Flax is an ingredient that I recommend you grind in small batches. You can use different appliances to grind flax seeds like a high-performance blender or food processor, but don't. You will end up with a lot more than you need with these machines. You should only grind what you'll use for a 2-week period of time, otherwise the oils in flax can go bad once exposed to oxygen.

For small quantities, I recommend using a coffee grinder that is dedicated to grinding herbs (not coffee beans) or a simple mortar and pestle. Store excess ground flax meal in an airtight container in the refrigerator or freezer.

Chickpea Veggie Skillet Bread

Makes 8–10 servings.

This is a healthier alternative to cornbread. I love it as an accompaniment to chili — either the meat or the vegetarian version. Yum!

Ingredients

1 Tbsp. coconut oil or avocado oil

½ onion, diced

1 bell pepper, seeded and diced

1 small, sweet potato, skin removed, grated

½ cup zucchini, diced

½ cup tomato, diced

½ cup sliced mushrooms

2–3 cloves garlic, minced

1¼ cup chickpea flour

¼ cup arrowroot powder

3 Tbsp. nutritional yeast

1 tsp. baking powder

1½ tsp. salt

½ tsp. black pepper

½ tsp. chili powder

½ tsp. smoked paprika

¼ tsp. cumin

1½ cups vegetable stock

Directions

Preheat oven to 350°F.

Generously butter or oil a 9" cast iron skillet or oven-proof sauté pan. Be sure to oil the sides. Add the diced onion, bell pepper, and sweet potato. Heat about 5 minutes to soften, stirring occasionally. Add in the zucchini, tomato, mushrooms, and garlic. Stir to combine for an additional 3–5 minutes, then remove from heat.

In a separate bowl, mix the chickpea flour, arrowroot powder, nutritional yeast, baking powder, and seasonings together. Add the stock and whisk together until smooth. Pour into the pan with the vegetables and mix.

Bake for approximately 35 minutes. The edges will be browned, and you will see cracks all over the surface when it is done. Serve warm.

Note

If you don't have an oven-proof skillet, you can use a small, oiled casserole dish or muffin tin with parchment liners instead.

Variations

- Substitute any of the vegetables with spinach, broccoli, etc.
- Nutritional yeast gives a delicious cheesy flavor and adds important B vitamins — all while avoiding dairy! If you don't have easy access to this product and digest dairy easily, just sprinkle some grated cheese instead.
- Add bacon or cooked pancetta.

Serving suggestions

This pairs well with **Everyone Loves Chili** (see page 51), a green salad, soup, or can be served on its own with some **Easy Guacamole** (see page 115).

Cheesy Herb Rolls

Makes 6 servings.

A savory bun that will satisfy your craving for bread. A nice addition to any soup, stew, or salad meal.

Ingredients

Coconut oil or avocado oil or cooking spray

¼ cup + 1 Tbsp. chickpea flour

½ tsp. baking soda

¼ tsp. salt

1 tsp. cream of tartar

¼ cup butter, cold or frozen

3 eggs

¼ cup fresh chopped herbs (parsley, cilantro, basil, etc.)

¼ cup coconut cream

½ cup freshly grated cheese of choice

Directions

Preheat oven to 450°F. Coat 6 spaces in a muffin/cupcake tray with oil or butter. Or, to keep cleanup simple, use paper baking cups.

Add the chickpea flour, baking soda, salt, and cream of tartar to a medium bowl. Mix to incorporate. Grate the cold butter on top of the flour mixture. Cut the butter in so it is crumbly and evenly coated.

In a separate bowl, whisk together the eggs, herbs, and coconut cream. Pour the wet ingredients over the butter/flour mixture and stir with a fork to combine. The mixture will be soupy. Let it stand for 5 minutes to thicken.

Pour the batter evenly into the prepared muffin tin pockets. Top each muffin batter with some grated cheese.

Bake in the oven 11–13 minutes or until golden and a toothpick inserted into the center comes out clean.

Let cool on a wire rack. Store extras in an airtight container in the refrigerator to warm later.

Serving suggestions

This low carb, gluten-free roll can be used in place of an English muffin, as a breakfast sandwich, or as the perfect accompaniment to soup for lunch or dinner.

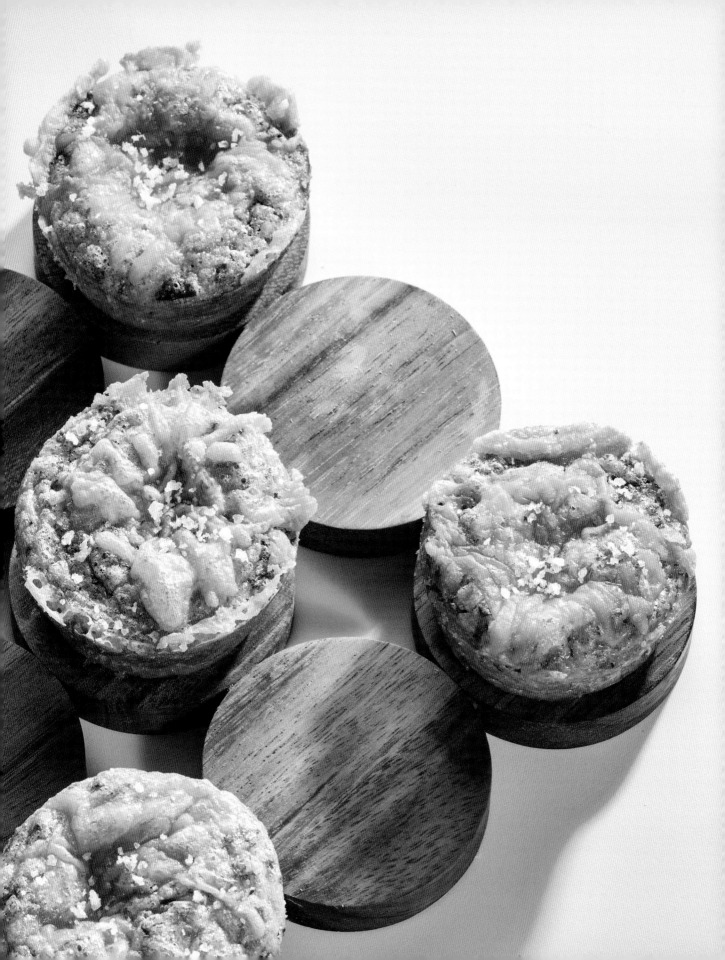

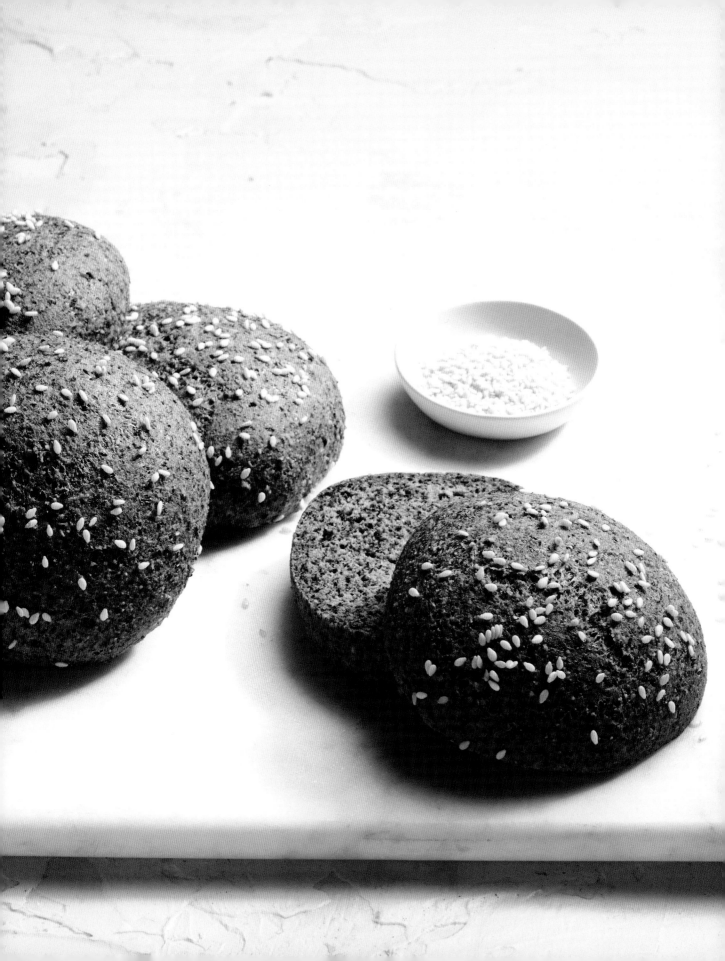

(You Don't Need a Lettuce Wrap) Burger Buns

Makes 4 regular-sized buns or 6 slider-sized buns.

Move over lettuce wraps; if you are looking to avoid bread, and are tired of lettuce, this recipe is your new best friend!

Ingredients

1¼ cups almond flour

2 Tbsp. psyllium husk powder

1 Tbsp. nutritional yeast

1 tsp. Italian herbs or paprika or chili powder (or choose your favorite seasoning)

1 tsp. baking soda

½ tsp. salt

3 egg whites

1 tsp. apple cider vinegar

⅔ cup boiling water

Directions

Preheat oven to 350°F. Line a baking tray with parchment paper.

In a medium bowl, combine the dry ingredients.

In a small bowl whisk together the egg whites and apple cider vinegar until frothy. Add egg/vinegar mixture to the dry ingredients. Mix using a handheld mixer or spatula. This will form a thick batter.

Pour in the hot water and stir quickly to incorporate it. This will make the dough easy to work with.

For regular size buns, divide the dough into four equal-sized portions. For sliders, make at least 6 portions. Shape into balls, place on the parchment, and flatten to roughly 1" thickness. The buns will double or more in size as they bake.

Bake 40–50 minutes. Let cool on a wire rack, then slice in half, across the middle, to use as a burger bun.

Note

Store any extras in an airtight container in the refrigerator and reheat to serve.

Serving suggestions

These buns are perfect for burgers, but you could use them for any type of sandwich or make them smaller for dinner rolls to go with soup or salad. They taste great toasted, too!

Garlic Greens

Makes 4 servings.

A tasty way to eat your greens every day!

Ingredients

6–8 cups fresh greens (try kale, spinach, chard, or a combination)

2 Tbsp. coconut oil or avocado oil

6–8 cloves garlic, minced, to taste

2–3 Tbsp. water

1 tsp. crushed red pepper flakes (optional)

½ tsp. salt

¼ tsp. black pepper

Optional garnishes

Parmesan cheese; or make **Dairy-free Parmesan Cheese** (see page 75)

Squeeze of fresh lemon juice

Directions

If you are using greens with sturdy stalks, like kale or collards, de-stem the greens. You can do this by holding the thick end of the stalk in one hand and running your other hand along the stem. This will strip the leaf from the base to the top. This step is not necessary for spinach, chard, or softer greens. After you have de-stemmed all greens, roll the leaves together and chop into smaller bite-sized ribbons.

Heat the oil in a saucepan over medium heat. Add the minced garlic and sauté for about 30 seconds, until fragrant.

Add the greens and water and stir continuously, about 1–2 minutes, until the ribbons start to wilt and turn bright green. Mix in the red pepper flakes.

Remove from heat. Season with salt and pepper and Parmesan cheese, or a squeeze of lemon, if desired. Serve immediately.

"Cheezy" Broccoli (Dairy-free)

Makes 4 servings.

This is a kid-friendly, tasty side dish. Nutritional yeast is the secret to creating the cheesy effect without the dairy!

Ingredients

- 1 head of broccoli
- Water
- 3 Tbsp., or more nutritional yeast
- Drizzle of olive oil, to taste
- Dash of salt, to taste

Directions

Cut the broccoli into bite-sized pieces. Steam for about 5 minutes in a steamer or large pot with a small amount of water, until just tender.

Remove from heat and sprinkle with a few tablespoons of nutritional yeast, a drizzle of olive oil, and some salt. Mix to combine evenly. Don't be afraid to use a generous amount of nutritional yeast. You want to create a definite taste effect. Taste and adjust flavors, as necessary, to create this cheese-like flavor.

Variation

Sprinkle a little cayenne powder or chili powder if you like it spicy!

Serving suggestions

Serve as a base, instead of rice, for any meal. Pairs well with **Curried Chicken Skillet** (see page 88) or **Garlic Shrimp** (see page 82).

Nutritional yeast (different from baker's yeast or brewer's yeast) is usually sold as thin, pale yellow flakes in a shaker bottle. You can find it in bulk bins in health food stores or in the spice/condiment section of the grocery.

Popular with vegans and vegetarians, nutritional yeast is rich in nutrients and has a savory, umami flavor. It's also free of soy, gluten, and sugar, making it a great addition for people who have food sensitivities.

Most nutritional yeast is especially rich in important B vitamins, including thiamine (B1), riboflavin (B2), niacin (B3), B6, and B12. It also contains zinc, selenium, molybdenum, and manganese, which are important for gene regulation, metabolism, immunity, and growth.

Marinated Mushrooms

Makes 4 servings.

These are delicious and versatile. They are a great side dish — or use as a topping with a warm or cold meal.

Ingredients

3 Tbsp. olive oil

1 Tbsp. lemon juice

2 tsp. tamari or nama shoyu

2 cloves garlic, minced

1 tsp. fresh parsley, minced

½ tsp. salt

2 cups fresh mushrooms, sliced

Directions

Combine olive oil, lemon juice, tamari, garlic, parsley, and salt. Add the sliced mushrooms and let marinate for an hour or more, stirring occasionally.

Drain the extra sauce from the mushrooms and reserve the liquid.

Note

The extra marinade stores well in the refrigerator for several days and can be used as a dressing for other salads or a marinade for fish or other dishes.

Beyond this recipe

You can use the marinated mushrooms in any recipe or salad for a boost of flavor. Try them in the **Cauliflower Quiche** (see page 33) and **Egg Florentine Breakfast Muffins** (see page 34).

· ·

Basic Cauliflower Rice

Makes 4-6 servings.

A versatile accompaniment to almost any meal when you want to avoid extra carbs. Use it anywhere you would normally have rice or other grains.

Ingredients

1 head cauliflower

1 Tbsp. coconut oil, avocado oil, or butter

1 tsp. salt

½ tsp. black pepper

Directions

Chop cauliflower into small chunks. Then use a food processor to grate the cauliflower into smaller, rice-sized pieces. You can do this by hand with a knife or grater, but a food processor will save time.

Heat a pan over medium-high heat. Add the oil or butter and the cauliflower. Cook for 5–8 minutes, stirring occasionally. Season to taste with salt, pepper, and any other seasoning you'd enjoy. Serve warm.

Cashew Sour Cream

Makes about 2 cups.

One of my favorite "go to" recipes for a topping sauce that is versatile and delicious with soups, entrees, and almost anything. It stores well in an airtight glass jar for a week or more in the fridge.

Ingredients

3 cups raw cashews

1 cup water (more or less, as necessary to achieve your desired consistency)

¼ cup lemon juice

1 Tbsp. apple cider vinegar

1 heaping tsp. salt

Directions

Blend all ingredients together in a food processor or high-performance blender until creamy. Add water, if needed, to blend more easily and to make a thinner consistency. If you like a stronger flavor, increase the lemon juice and/or the apple cider vinegar, to taste.

This dairy-free sour cream goes well with tacos, burgers, as a garnish for soups, or anywhere you would use regular dairy sour cream.

Note

If you don't have a strong food processor or blender, you can soak the cashews an hour or two ahead of time to soften and make them easier to blend.

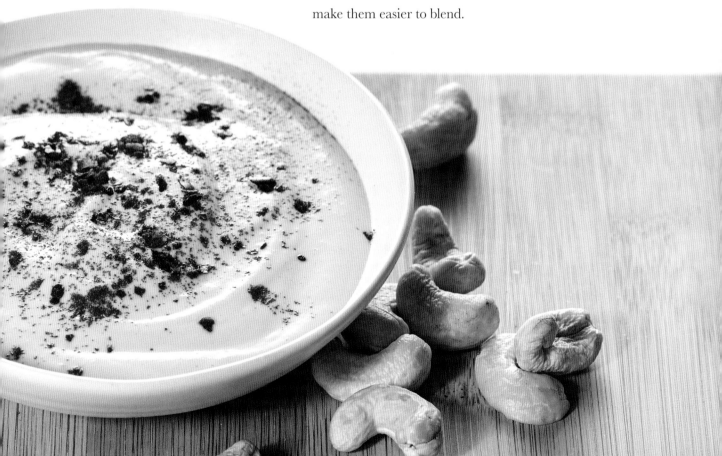

Easy Coconut Yogurt

Makes 1–2 servings.

Add some healthy probiotics to your inner ecosystem. Your body will thank you!

Ingredients

Fresh or defrosted coconut meat from
1 young Thai coconut (about 1 cup)

½–1 cup coconut water

2 capsules probiotic powder

Directions

Blend the coconut meat with the coconut water in a high-performance blender until smooth, and you have a yogurt-like texture. Start with less, then add more coconut water, if needed, to achieve your desired consistency.

Pour into a very clean glass jar with a lid. Open the probiotic powder capsules and empty the contents into the jar with the blended coconut. Stir to mix. Let sit to ferment, loosely covered, on the counter for 20–24 hours. The yogurt will begin to bubble slightly. And, it will taste a bit tart, as it ferments.

Store in the refrigerator, where it will continue to ferment, but at a slower pace.

Note

The ambient temperature in the room will affect how quickly the yogurt ferments. It will happen quicker in warmer weather. Allow for this and taste test your yogurt at different intervals until you achieve your ideal fermentation.

Variation

Blend in any flavors (fresh or dried fruits, cinnamon, or vanilla extract), if desired. Enjoy this yogurt like you would any type of yogurt. Consume within 4 days.

Coconut yogurt is a versatile and healthy food that vegans, and people who are sensitive to dairy, will find useful and delicious. Coconut yogurt is free from lactose and casein, which can cause digestive issues in some people. It is naturally creamy and sweet. Homemade coconut yogurt contains a lot more nutrition than store-bought varieties. Fermented coconut yogurt is a probiotic-rich food that is packed with good bacteria that can support the digestive system.

Spicy Garlic Tomato Sauce

Makes about a cup.

A versatile condiment sauce that's easy to make.

Ingredients

- 2 cups cherry tomatoes
- 1 Tbsp. avocado oil
- 2 cloves garlic, minced
- 2 Tbsp. balsamic vinegar
- 1–2 tsp. fresh thyme
- 1 Tbsp. butter
- ¼ tsp. paprika
- Salt and black pepper, to taste
- Dash of chili powder or cayenne pepper (optional)

Directions

In a dry sauté pan over high heat, cook the cherry tomatoes until the skins start to blister. Once they get a little soft, you can turn the heat down and add the avocado oil and garlic.

Smash the tomatoes gently with the back of a spoon, so they release their juices. Add the balsamic vinegar and thyme, and let the mixture reduce and thicken on low heat.

After 5–10 minutes, your sauce should be ready. Add the butter and paprika. Season with salt, pepper, and chili powder.

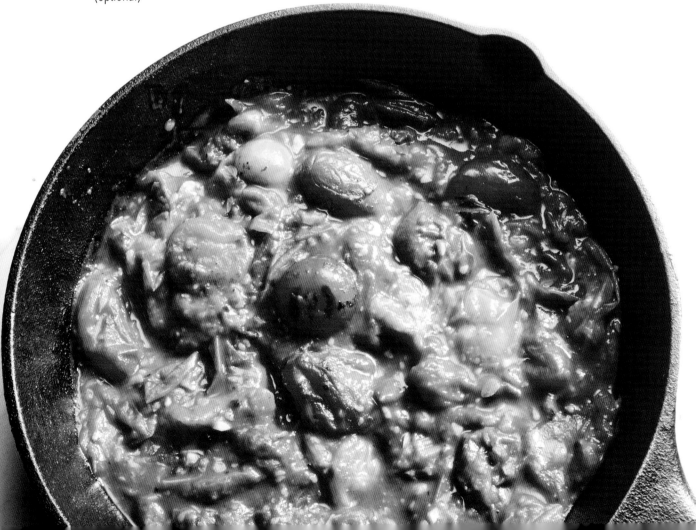

Yam Veggie Hash

Serves 4.

This is a delicious side dish that can be enjoyed with meat or fish of your choice, or as its own meal. Yams are a tuber rich in vitamins, minerals, and fiber. Combining it with other vegetables lowers the glycemic index even more!

Ingredients

- 2 Tbsp. coconut oil or butter
- 1 small red onion, chopped
- 3 cloves garlic, minced
- 2 lbs. yams (about 3 medium or 2 large), peeled
- 1 red pepper, seeded and diced
- ½ cup mushrooms, chopped
- Pinch of chili powder
- Pinch of paprika
- Salt and black pepper to taste
- Egg wash (1 egg or egg substitute, beaten with a tablespoon of water)

Directions

Grate the yams using the standard large holes in a grater.

In a large skillet over medium-high heat, add the oil and the onions and sauté for a couple minutes to soften the onions slowly. Then add in the garlic, grated yams, diced pepper and chopped mushrooms. Season with chili, paprika, salt and pepper.

Continue to sauté for 10–15 minutes until vegetables are tender and onions are translucent. Transfer the mixture to a greased baking pan and brush with the egg wash.

Bake for about 15–20 minutes at 375°F or broil for five minutes, until yam hash is browned on top and you have reached your desired level of crispiness.

Yams and sweet potatoes are often used interchangeably, but sweet potato refers to the vegetables with smooth, reddish skin and orange flesh (though they can also be white), while yams have a rough brown skin and are more of an off-white color with a starchy taste. True yams are closer in flavor to the yucca plant than sweet potatoes. Sweet potatoes contain more carbs, so yams may be a healthier choice for people who are concerned about high blood sugar and Type 2 diabetes. However, some markets may label sweet potatoes as yams and true yams can be hard to find, so ask your grocer to be sure.

Spicy Low-Carb Squash Casserole

Serves 4–6.

While it's fine to enjoy a small amount of sweet potatoes every now and then, why not reduce the glycemic load even more and substitute butternut squash? Including cauliflower reduces the carbs even further, and the final product is a perfect taste alternative to the real thing.

Ingredients

Casserole

5 cups butternut squash peeled and cubed

3 cups cauliflower florets

2 Tbsp. butter, melted

½-1 tsp cumin

½ tsp cinnamon

Pinch of nutmeg

Pinch of cayenne and/or chili powder

Salt and pepper to taste

1 Tbsp. maple syrup

Topping

¾ cup pecans or spicy pecans, chopped

2 Tbsp. coconut or date sugar

3 Tbsp. butter melted

½ tsp. cinnamon

Directions

Preheat the oven to 400°F. Prepare a baking tray lined with parchment and a greased loaf tin.

Spread the butternut squash and cauliflower onto the baking tray, and bake for 30 minutes, then remove from oven and cool.

Add the cooled vegetables to a food processor or blender with the rest of the seasonings, maple syrup and butter. Blend until smooth. Layer the mixture into the bottom of a greased loaf pan or small casserole dish.

Add the topping ingredients to a mixing bowl, and stir to combine well. Crumble the topping over the pureed mixture. Bake for 20 minutes.

Note

Here is a great opportunity to add some of those beneficial spices into the mix to support healthy circulation and metabolism at the same time!

Tahini Dressing

Makes 4-6 servings.

A tasty sauce that can be used on raw or steamed vegetables or any salad.

Ingredients

½ cup raw sesame tahini

½ cup water (or less)

¼ cup lemon juice

2 cloves garlic, peeled

¼ tsp. ground cumin

1 tsp. salt

Pinch of cayenne pepper

Directions

Place all ingredients in a blender. Blend until smooth. For a thicker sauce or dip, reduce the amount of water.

Note

You can store the dressing in the refrigerator in a sealed glass jar. It will keep for 3–5 days.

Serving suggestion

This is a delicious topper for the **Keto Macro Bowl** (see page 76).

Beyond this recipe

Use this spread to replace mayonnaise in a sandwich or salad. You will still get the richness, but it will add a subtle sesame flavor.

. . . .

Fresh Tomato Salsa

Makes about 2½ cups.

Salsa is an ideal low-carb snack you can enjoy with fresh vegetables or grain-free/low carb crackers. You can also add it as a garnish or flavor enhancer to many meals. Here's a salsa recipe you can use as-is or vary according to your taste.

Ingredients

2 cups tomatoes, diced

½ red onion, finely diced

½ cup fresh cilantro, chopped (optional)

1 jalapeño pepper, de-seeded and finely minced

2 cloves garlic, minced

½ tsp. salt

Juice of 1 lime

Directions

Mix ingredients together in a bowl and let marinate for an hour or two to let the flavors fuse. Or serve right away if you're short on time.

Easy Guacamole

Makes about 2 cups.

Ingredients

2–3 avocados, skin and pits removed

¾ cup of salsa; or make **Fresh Tomato Salsa** (see page 114)

Garlic, minced, to taste

Lime juice, to taste

Salt and black pepper, to taste

Directions

Mash avocados and mix in with the salsa.

If you decide to make a batch of **Fresh Tomato Salsa**, you can save about half of it to keep as salsa and use the other half as a base for this guacamole.

Taste and adjust with garlic, lime, salt, and pepper.

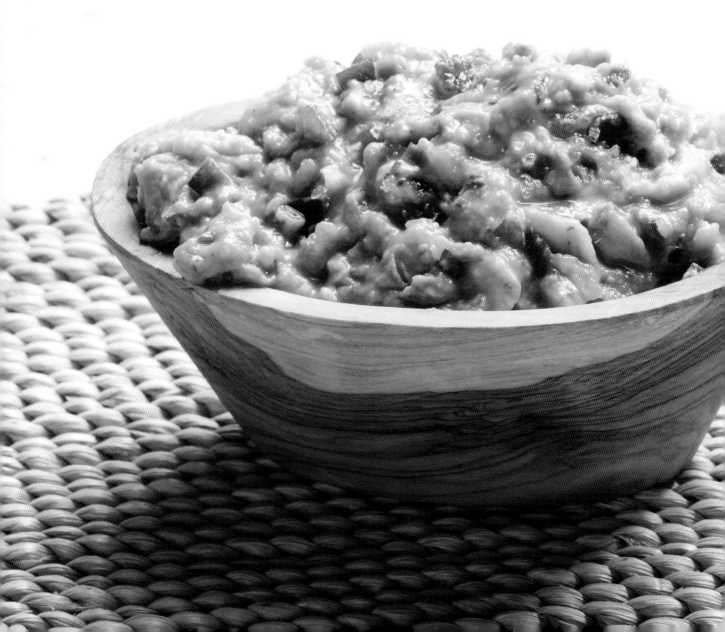

These next "warm" dressings were created by a friend of Dr. John, Diya Loney. The theory for these dressings is that most people use cold, refrigerated dressings to pour over and flavor salads. These dressings often contain an abundance of salt, added as a flavor enhancer and preservative for increasing the product's shelf life. However, I suggest you can enhance the flavor of your salads and vegetable dishes with a healthier, warm, spicy dressing instead.

You can also use these warm dressings on a variety of different vegetables and legumes. They truly add more enjoyment to your dining experience and might encourage you to choose vegetables more often. Pour a warm dressing over a fresh salad, steamed vegetables, cooked legumes, baked potatoes, or yams.

Most of these recipes can be made on a stove top or in an instant pot. They can all be frozen and saved in a freezer-safe, airtight container for up to one month. The ideal way to defrost them is to move the container from the freezer into the refrigerator and leave it there for 12 to 24 hours. Once it has defrosted in the fridge, it can be heated in the microwave. Enjoy!

Roasted Tomato Warm, Spicy Dressing

Makes 3 cups.

This is both a dressing and a soup. You know it's special, since it's good enough to eat on its own!

Ingredients

10 Roma tomatoes, diced into 1" chunks

1 medium-sized onion, diced into 1" chunks

3 garlic cloves, whole

3 Tbsp. olive oil

1 tsp. chili flakes

¼ cup basil leaves

¼ cup parsley

2 tsp. fresh rosemary, or 1 tsp. dried

1 Tbsp. balsamic vinegar

1 Tbsp. brown sugar

1½ cups low-sodium broth (chicken, bone, or vegetable)

Salt, to taste

Directions

Preheat oven to 450°F. Line a 9" x 13" sheet pan with parchment paper.

Scatter the tomatoes, onions, and garlic on the pan. Coat with the olive oil and chili flakes. Roast the mixture, stirring every 10 minutes. Cook for about 30 minutes, or until the onions and tomatoes are done to your liking.

Put the roasted mixture into a blender. Add the basil, parsley, rosemary, balsamic vinegar, brown sugar, and broth. Blend until smooth. Taste for seasoning. Adjust and add salt, if needed.

Pour into a saucepan and heat on medium-low until it boils. Enjoy warm as a soup or as a dressing for salads, roasted vegetables, etc.

Warm, Spicy Dal Dressing

Makes 3 cups.

This can be made mild or spicy. Feel free to adjust the spices according to your taste and preferences.

Ingredients

  1 cup dry red lentils

  3 cups water, plus more for rinsing and soaking, divided

  1 Tbsp. neutral oil (like grapeseed or avocado oil)

  ½ tsp. cumin seeds

  1 tsp. fresh ginger, finely chopped

  1 large clove garlic, finely chopped

  ¼ tsp. turmeric

  ½ tsp. cayenne pepper

  ¼ tsp. coriander

  ¼ tsp. garam masala

  2 Tbsp. tomato paste

  1 tsp. salt, or to taste

Stovetop Directions

Rinse the lentils with water, until the water runs clear. Then cover them with fresh water and soak for about 30 minutes to an hour. Set aside.

In a large pot over medium heat, add the oil and cumin seeds. Sauté until the seeds start sizzling. Stir in the chopped ginger and garlic. Sauté until fragrant and lightly browned.

Add the rest of the dried spices and sauté for a few more seconds. Spoon in the tomato paste and stir to incorporate.

Drain the soaking water from the lentils. Spoon the lentils into the pot with the other ingredients, along with 3 cups water. Mix and bring to a boil. Then lower the heat, cover, and simmer—stirring occasionally—until the lentils are tender, about 20 to 30 minutes.

If desired, purée for a creamy texture, using an immersion or traditional blender.

Taste and add salt, if needed.

Instant pot directions

Start the instant pot in sauté mode and let it heat up. Add all in the ingredients, except the salt, following the stovetop directions.

Pressure cook for 15 minutes at high pressure. Wait for the pressure to release naturally. Open the instant pot.

Mix well. Taste and add salt, if needed.

Variation

If you like additional spice and heat, try this additional step called *tadka*, or tempering. In a small saucepan, heat 1 tsp. ghee, or any neutral-flavored oil and cumin seeds. Sauté until ¼ tsp. cumin seeds start sizzling. Add the ¼–½ tsp. cayenne pepper and sauté for a few seconds. Pour this spicy combination over your dal dressing and mix it in.

Miso and Squash Warm, Spicy Dressing

Makes 3½ to 4 cups.

This is a delicious way to incorporate squash into your diet. No need to salt this dressing, since miso, broth, and soy sauce are all sources of salt.

Ingredients

- 1 tsp. toasted sesame oil
- 1 Tbsp. neutral oil (like grapeseed or avocado oil)
- ½ medium onion, thinly sliced
- 1 large clove garlic, finely chopped
- 1 tsp. fresh ginger, finely chopped
- ¼ tsp. turmeric, or to taste
- ¼ tsp. cumin, or to taste
- ½ tsp. cayenne pepper, or to taste
- ½ tsp. black pepper, or to taste
- ½ lb. squash, peeled and cubed (acorn, butternut, delicata, kabocha)
- 2 cups low-sodium broth (chicken, bone, or vegetable)
- 1 Tbsp. tomato paste
- 1 Tbsp. red or white miso paste
- 2 tsp. soy sauce

Stovetop Directions

Combine both oils in a large pot over medium heat. Stir in the sliced onions and sauté until they begin to caramelize.

Add the chopped garlic and ginger. Mix well and cook for about 30 seconds. Stir in the rest of the dried spices and sauté for another 30 seconds.

Add the cubed squash, broth, tomato paste and miso paste. Mix well and bring to a boil. Then lower the heat, cover the pot and simmer—stirring occasionally—until the squash is tender, about 20 minutes. Add the soy sauce and stir to combine.

Purée the sauce, using an immersion or traditional blender.

Instant pot directions

Start the instant pot in sauté mode and let it heat up.

Add in all the ingredients, except the soy sauce, following the stovetop directions.

Pressure cook for 10 minutes at high pressure. Wait for the pressure to release naturally.

Open the instant pot. Add the soy sauce and stir to combine.

Warm, Spicy Onion Dressing

Makes about 3 cups.

Like a French onion soup for your salad — minus all the unhealthy ingredients.

Ingredients

2 Tbsp. butter

1½ lbs red or yellow onions (not sweet onions), thinly sliced

¼ tsp. salt

2 cups low-sodium beef broth (or any low-sodium broth or water)

1 tsp. white or red miso paste

1 tsp. black pepper, to taste

½ tsp. cayenne pepper, to taste

1 tsp. soy sauce

Stovetop Directions

In a large pot over medium heat, sauté the butter, onions, and salt together. Stir every few minutes, until the onions are caramelized and golden brown. This can take up to 30 minutes, depending on the moisture content of the onions.

Deglaze the pan, using the beef broth. A lot of flavor lives in those browned bits stuck to the bottom. You'll want to get all of those off the pan and integrated back into the liquid.

Stir in the miso paste and dry spices and mix well. Bring to a boil, then lower the heat, cover and simmer — stirring occasionally — until the onions are tender, about 20 minutes. Add the soy sauce and stir to combine.

Purée the sauce, using an immersion or traditional blender. Or, you could leave this dressing chunky, if you like the texture.

Instant pot directions

Start the instant pot in sauté mode on high and let it heat up.

Add all in the ingredients, except the soy sauce, following the stovetop directions.

Cover and pressure cook on high for 5 minutes. Wait for the pressure to release naturally.

Open the instant pot. Add the soy sauce and stir to combine.

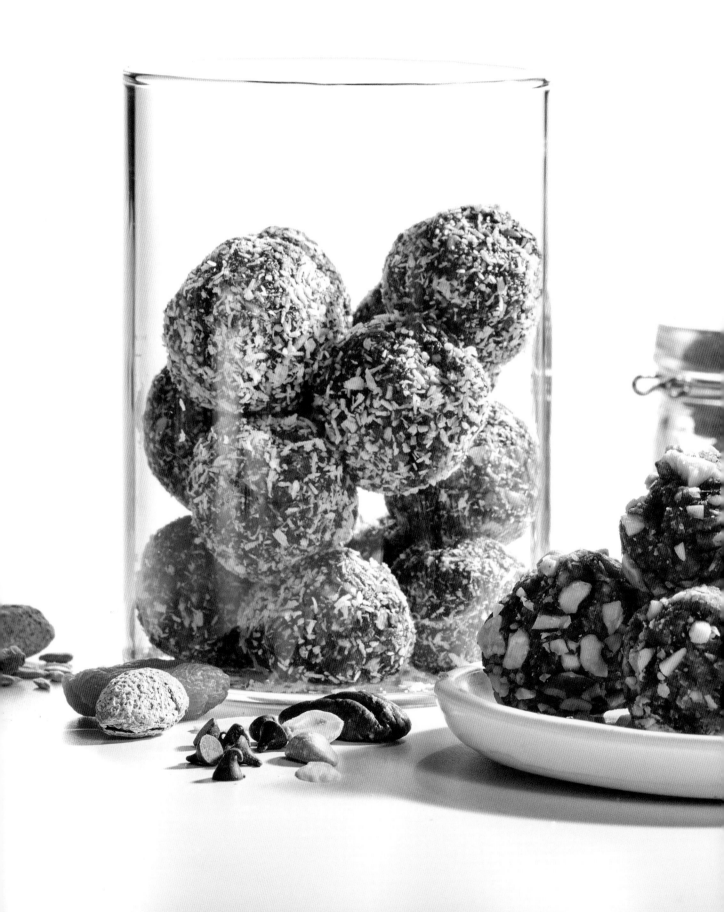

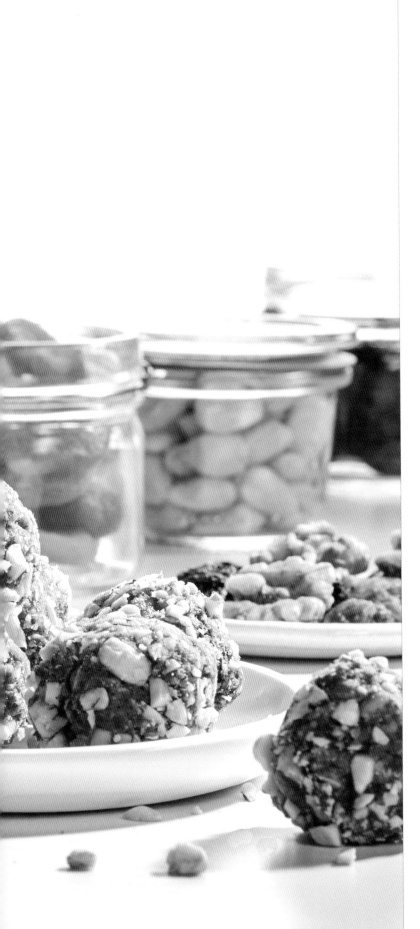

DESSERTS

Moist Chocolate Cake with Avocado Icing

Makes 12 slices.

This cake is grain-free, gluten-free, dairy-free, vegetarian, and refined-sugar-free. It's ideal for special occasions and is a healthier addition to any dessert table. The use of black beans will give you a nutritive boost without compromising texture or flavor.

Ingredients

Cake

- 1 medium ripe banana
- 1 15-oz. can black beans (1½ cups fresh), drained and rinsed
- 5 large eggs
- 4 tsp. vanilla extract
- ½ tsp. sea salt
- 3 Tbsp. coconut oil, melted
- ½ cup unsweetened cocoa baking powder, or raw cacao powder
- 2 tsp. baking soda
- 2 tsp. apple cider vinegar
- ¼ cup coconut or date sugar

Icing

- 2 medium avocados, peeled and pits removed
- 1 Tbsp. lemon juice
- ¼ cup honey or real maple syrup (not pancake syrup)
- ¼ cup unsweetened cocoa baking powder, or raw cacao powder
- Pinch of salt

Optional garnishes

- Shredded coconut
- Fresh berries
- Fresh mint leaves
- Coconut whip cream

Directions

Preheat oven to 325°F. Prepare an 8" or 9" baking pan: oil or line with parchment paper.

Cake

Mash the banana in a medium mixing bowl. Set aside.

Combine the remaining cake ingredients in a blender or food processor, and blend until smooth. Transfer the batter into the bowl with the banana. Mix until evenly incorporated.

Pour into the prepared pan. Bake for 40 minutes. Cake is done when the top is rounded and firm to the touch and an inserted toothpick comes out clean. Let cool on a wire rack, then remove from pan.

For best results, refrigerate for at least 1–2 hours to chill — or overnight, if you have time.

Icing

Place avocados in a mixing bowl and add lemon juice. Use a hand mixer to blend to a smooth consistency. Add sweetener, cocoa powder, and salt, and continue to mix until smooth and creamy. Taste and adjust for desired sweetness.

Assemble

Frost the cake just before serving and garnish as you'd like.

Notes

- This recipe can be made as cupcakes in a muffin tin. Reduce the baking time by about 10 minutes.
- Store leftover icing/cake in the refrigerator for up to a week.

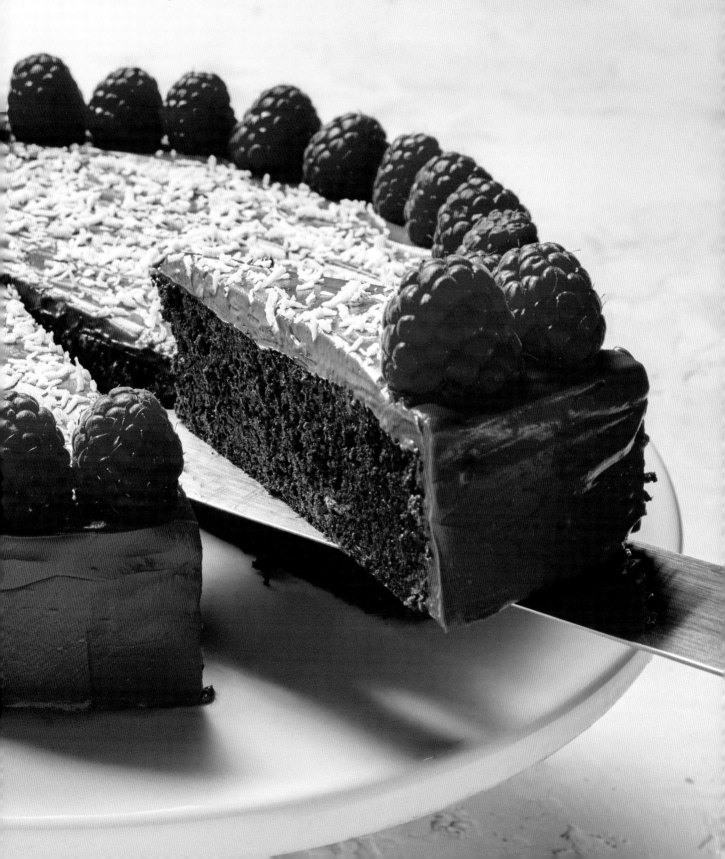

Chock full of black beans and avocados—your guests will never guess!

Amazing Quinoa Brownies

Makes 12-16 squares.

Who says you can't enjoy dessert? These amazing protein-packed brownies will satisfy any craving for a sweet treat.

Ingredients

- ¾ cup raw cacao powder
- ⅔ cup quinoa flour
- ½ cup coconut sugar
- ⅓ cup date sugar, to taste
- ⅓ cup coconut oil, melted to liquid state
- 1 small banana, mashed
- 6 Tbsp. chia seeds, freshly ground in a coffee grinder or high performance blender
- ¾ tsp. salt
- ½ tsp. baking soda
- ½ tsp. baking powder
- 2-4 Tbsp. water, as needed
- ½ cup dark, or low sugar, chocolate chips (optional)

Directions

Preheat the oven to 350°F. Prepare an 8" x 8" baking pan: oil and line with parchment paper.

Mix all the ingredients (except chocolate chips) together in a bowl. Start with just a small amount of the date sugar, adding more only if needed, according to your palate. (Since there are no eggs in this batter, it's safe to taste the batter, to test for sweetness.)

Add a small amount of water to make a nice, substantial batter. The batter should be thick, but not so thick that it is difficult to transfer evenly to the baking pan. After you are happy with your batter, then add chocolate chips for extra chocolate richness!

Bake approximately 30 minutes, until a toothpick comes out clean. These brownies are gluten-free and dairy-free (if no chocolate chips are used).

Decadent, Raw Chocolate Pudding

Makes 4 servings.

A fan favorite. It's easy to make and stores well in the fridge, but no one will let it sit there for long!

Ingredients

2 ripe avocados, peeled and pitted

¾ cup raw cacao powder

½ cup coconut nectar, coconut sugar, or real maple syrup (not pancake syrup)

¾ cup coconut oil

½ cup coconut water

1 tsp. vanilla extract

⅛ tsp. salt

Optional garnishes

Fresh berries, to taste

Fresh mint leaves, to taste

Coconut whip cream

Directions

Combine all ingredients in a food processor or high-performance blender. Process until smooth. Taste and adjust for sweetness. You can make the pudding thinner and lighter by adding more coconut water. Make it thicker and fudgier by using more coconut oil, which will harden when chilled.

Spoon into individual serving dishes and chill in the refrigerator for at least 1–2 hours. The mixture will thicken as it chills.

Serve topped with a garnish of fresh berries and/or mint leaves and some coconut whipped cream.

Note

This pudding will keep up to one week in the refrigerator.

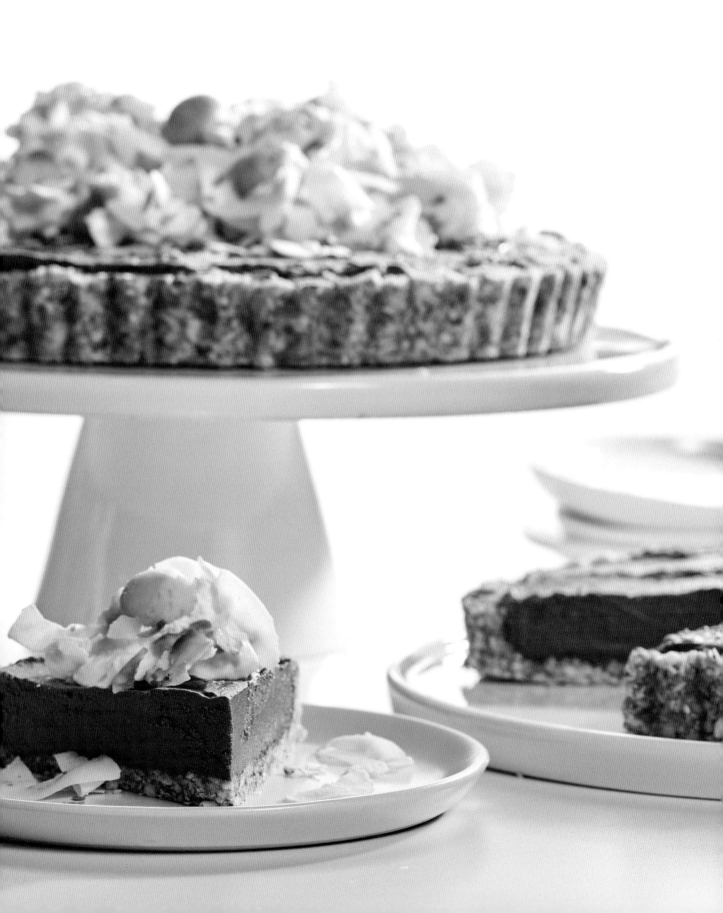

Mocha Torte with Coconut Crust

Makes 8-12 servings.

This is decadent treat. The fudge-like filling is rich and reminds me of a European pastry. It's pretty, too!

Ingredients

Crust

1 cup raw almonds, pecans, or macadamia nuts

1 cup shredded unsweetened coconut

½ cup medjool dates, pitted, plus more if needed

1 tsp. vanilla extract

½ tsp. cinnamon

Pinch of salt

Dash of cayenne pepper

1-2 Tbsp. coconut oil, as needed

Filling

5 ripe avocados, peeled and pitted

1¾ cups raw cacao powder

¾ cup coconut nectar or coconut sugar

1 cup coconut oil, melted

1 cup coconut water

2 tsp. vanilla extract

¼ tsp. salt

1-2 Tbsp. instant espresso powder or coffee substitute (see note)

Optional garnishes

Coconut whipped cream, to taste

Shredded coconut, to taste

Fresh berries, to taste

Pistachios, to taste

Directions

Crust

Prepare an 8" pie pan with coconut oil.

In a food processor, combine the nuts, dried coconut, dates, vanilla, salt, cinnamon, salt, and pepper. The ingredients should just start to stick together when pressed between your fingers. If the batter seems dry, add a tablespoon or two of melted coconut oil and/or 1 or 2 more dates.

Press the crust mixture evenly into the prepared pan, making sure it is consistently pressed around the edges. The crust should stick together and not be loose. Put in the refrigerator to set while you make the filling.

Filling

Combine all ingredients in a food processor or high-performance blender. Process until smooth. Stop the machine periodically and scrape down the sides of the container, so the texture will be consistent.

You can make the pudding thinner, as desired, by adding more coconut water. Remember, the filling will get more dense when it's refrigerated, because the coconut oil will solidify. Taste and adjust flavor, before assembling.

Assemble

Fill the crust with the pudding mixture and refrigerate, or freeze, to set. If frozen, allow at least 90 minutes for the pie to thaw before cutting. To serve, garnish with coconut whipped cream, shredded coconut and/or berries and pistachios.

Note

One tablespoon of espresso powder will enhance the chocolate flavor, while two will give the torte its distinct mocha taste. Also, you can swap out the espresso powder for an herbal coffee substitute, such as Dandy Blend.

No-Bake Haystack Cookies

Makes 10-12 cookies.

These are so much tastier than the cloyingly sweet version that many of us grew up with. The silhouette is a familiar, barnyard shape, but the flavor is all grown up!

Ingredients

⅓ cup medjool dates, pitted

⅓ cup coconut cream

8 Tbsp. butter

1 cup chopped pecans or walnuts

½–1 cup unsweetened coconut flakes or shreds

½–1 cup your favorite grain-free/high protein cereal

Optional garnishes

⅛ cup dark chocolate/low sugar chocolate chips

Dried fruit such as cranberries or raisins, to taste

Directions

Line a baking tray with parchment paper.

In a food processor or high-performance blender, combine the dates and coconut cream. (Check the dates before blending—if they do not feel soft enough to blend smoothly, you can soak them in water, in advance. Make sure the pits are removed and drain the water before blending.)

Put the butter in a saucepan over medium heat and melt gently. Add the date-cream mixture to the melted butter and combine. Stir constantly to avoid burning. When it starts bubbling, remove from heat and add the rest of the ingredients. The texture will be somewhat coarse.

Let cool slightly, then, using a spoon, drop 10–12 little 2" haystacks onto the prepared parchment paper.

If you want, you can sprinkle some chocolate chips or dried fruit on top of each cookie. Lightly press any garnishes into the haystacks and make sure they are the shape you want.

Place the tray of cookies into the refrigerator or freezer for 30–60 minutes to let harden.

Store in an airtight container in the refrigerator or freezer.

Note

There are many varieties of grain-free breakfast cereals available on the market. Look for something high in protein, low in carbs, and naturally sweetened. My favorite is "Catalina Crunch" which is made primarily from pea protein and comes in many varieties.

Variation

For a crunchier cookie, you can use coconut sugar instead of the dates. Just be aware of the carb count and perhaps add more shredded coconut and/or cereal to balance the protein and fiber.

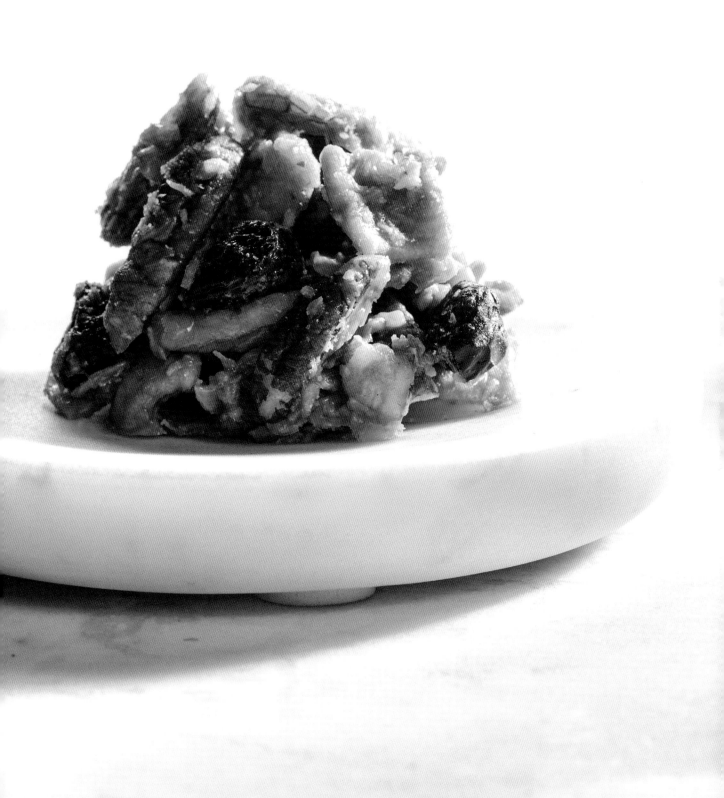

Refrigerator Chocolate-Dipped Macaroons

Makes 12 servings.

A wholesome treat that is helpful to have on standby when you want something sweet and delicious.

Ingredients

½ cup raw almonds (or almond flour)

1½ cups shredded coconut, unsweetened

½ cup raw cacao powder

¼ cup coconut butter (this is the coconut meat blended with oil, not just coconut oil)

½ cup raw organic honey, coconut nectar, or real maple syrup (not pancake syrup)

1 tsp. vanilla extract

Pinch of salt

4 oz. dark, or low sugar, chocolate

2–3 Tbsp. coconut oil (optional)

Directions

Line a baking tray with parchment paper.

If using raw almonds, place them in a food processor and grind them until they are finely chopped.

Add the shredded coconut to the ground almonds (or almond flour), along with the cacao powder, coconut butter, sweetener, vanilla extract, and salt. Process in the food processor until the mixture is well-blended but is not completely smooth.

Using a mini ice cream scoop, or tablespoon, scoop the mixture into balls. If very sticky, you can roll the balls in any extra shredded coconut. If not sticky enough, add a little coconut oil. Place the macaroons on the prepared baking tray and refrigerate to set.

When the macaroons are set (and cold), melt the dark chocolate in a double boiler over low heat. Make sure you don't get any water in the pot or the chocolate won't set properly. If your chocolate starts to seize, mix in a little coconut oil in to smooth it out.

Dip the bottom of each macaroon in the melted chocolate, and place back on the parchment sheet, chocolate side down, then back in the refrigerator. Serve at room temperature.

Note

Coconut oil will harden in the fridge and help give a nice shell to your macaroon.

Dairy-Free Lemon Pudding

Makes 2–3 servings.

Sweet and sour; a tangy alternative to chocolate.

Ingredients

1 cup Brazil nuts, soaked overnight

8 medjool dates, pitted and soaked, if necessary

¼ cup coconut cream; or make **Easy Coconut Yogurt** (see page 110)

Juice of 2 large or 3 small lemons

1 tsp. lemon peel

1 tsp. vanilla extract

Pinch of salt

Directions

Take the soaked Brazil nuts (and dates), and strain the liquid, but reserve it in case you need to adjust consistency in the pudding.

Process all ingredients in a food processor or high-performance blender until creamy. Add a little of the water used to soak the nuts and dates, if needed, to make blending easier.

Taste and adjust for tartness/sweetness. Add some lemon juice to make the pudding more tart or 1 or 2 dates to make it sweeter.

Note

You can pre-soak the nuts and dates together in the same bowl, overnight or for a few hours in advance to make them softer.

Serving suggestion

Top with **Mixed Berry Compote** (see page 31), or fresh fruit.

If you use a fermented coconut yogurt in this recipe, not only will it provide a tangier flavor, but you'll also get the probiotic benefits. You can buy the yogurt readymade or ferment your own for maximum digestive health. The coconut cream option will not provide the same health benefits as the fermented coconut yogurt, but it will give the pudding a nice creamy consistency.

You can try this icing on any low carb, gluten-free dessert, cake, cookie, or even a sweet potato. It's simple to make and will store well in the fridge for weeks.

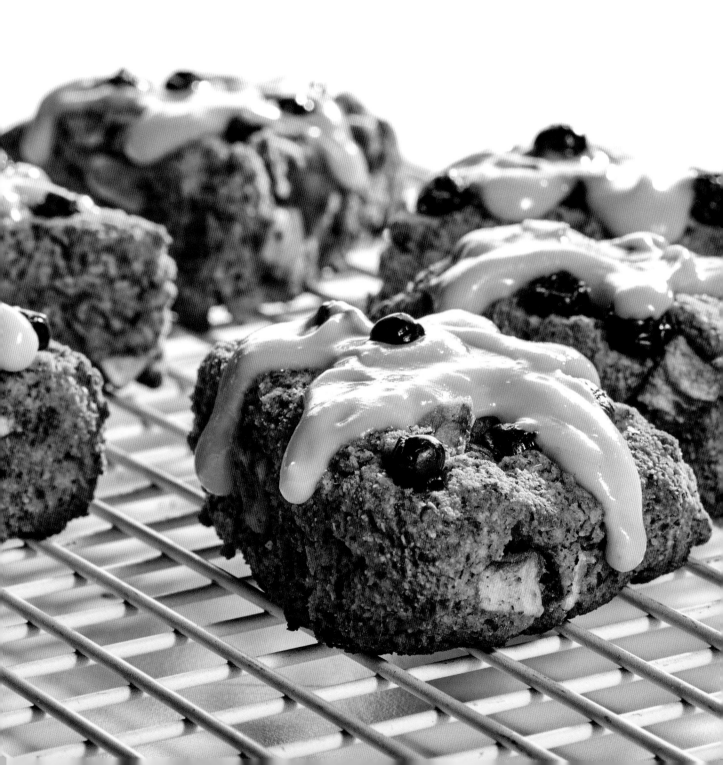

Apple-Ginger Gluten-Free "Scones" with Cashew Cream Icing

Makes 6 scones.

When you want a sweet treat with your afternoon tea. Cheers!

Ingredients

Icing

1 cup raw cashews

Water

¼ cup full-fat coconut milk or cream or yogurt

¼ cup coconut oil, melted

3–4 Tbsp. real maple syrup (not pancake syrup)

1–2 Tbsp. lemon juice

¼ tsp. lemon zest

1 tsp. pure vanilla extract

Pinch of salt

Scones

1½ cups almond flour (or ground almonds)

1 tsp. cinnamon

1 tsp. ginger powder

tsp. baking soda

⅛ tsp. sea salt

2 Tbsp. honey

1½ tsp. apple cider vinegar

2 tsp. freshly grated ginger

1 egg

1 medium apple, core removed, finely diced

¼ cup raisins or dried blueberries (optional)

Directions

Icing

Soak the cashews in hot water for at least an hour, to soften. (Or, soak in cold water for 4 or more hours.)

Drain cashews thoroughly and place all icing ingredients in a high-performance blender to make a smooth consistency. Blend until creamy, scraping down the sides, as needed. Taste and adjust flavors as desired. (Add more maple syrup for sweetness, lemon or apple cider vinegar for tanginess, or vanilla and salt for overall flavor.)

Chill in the refrigerator or freezer while you make the scones. The coconut oil will solidify, making the icing thicker and easier to spread.

Scones

Preheat oven to 375°F. Line a baking tray with parchment paper.

Add all dry ingredients in a bowl and mix with a fork until well combined.

In a separate bowl, mix the honey, apple cider vinegar, fresh ginger, and egg together.

Pour the wet ingredients mixture into dry ingredients and stir until just combined. Add the chopped apples and make sure they are evenly distributed.

Pack the dough gently into one big ball, then flatten into a disc shape, about 1" high. Slice the disc into 6 wedges. Top with a sprinkle of raisins or dried.

With a spatula, gently transfer each wedge to the baking tray. Bake approximately 15 minutes until lightly browned.

Assemble

Allow scones to cool fully. Top with **Cashew Cream Icing.**

Nutty Chickpea Cookie Dough Bliss Balls

Makes about 12 servings.

Bliss Balls are a cross between a cookie and a high-protein power bar. These little orbs of energy are perfect for a hike, or for an afternoon snack when you need a pick-me-up.

Ingredients

- 1 15-oz. can chickpeas (or 1½ cups cooked), rinsed and drained
- ½ cup almond flour
- ½ cup macaroon-style shredded coconut, unsweetened
- ⅓ cup your favorite nut butter or sunflower seed butter
- ¼ cup dried cranberries
- 2 Tbsp. coconut or date sugar
- 2 tsp. vanilla
- 1 tsp. cinnamon
- Pinch salt
- ½ cup finely chopped nuts of choice (pecans are great)

Directions

Line a baking tray with parchment paper.

Combine all ingredients, except the chopped nuts, in a medium-sized mixing bowl. Stir dough completely.

Place the nuts in a small bowl. Use a spoon to scoop the dough into balls approximately 1" in size, then roll in the finely crushed nuts to coat your Bliss Balls completely.

Refrigerate the Bliss Balls to set. Serve chilled or room temperature.

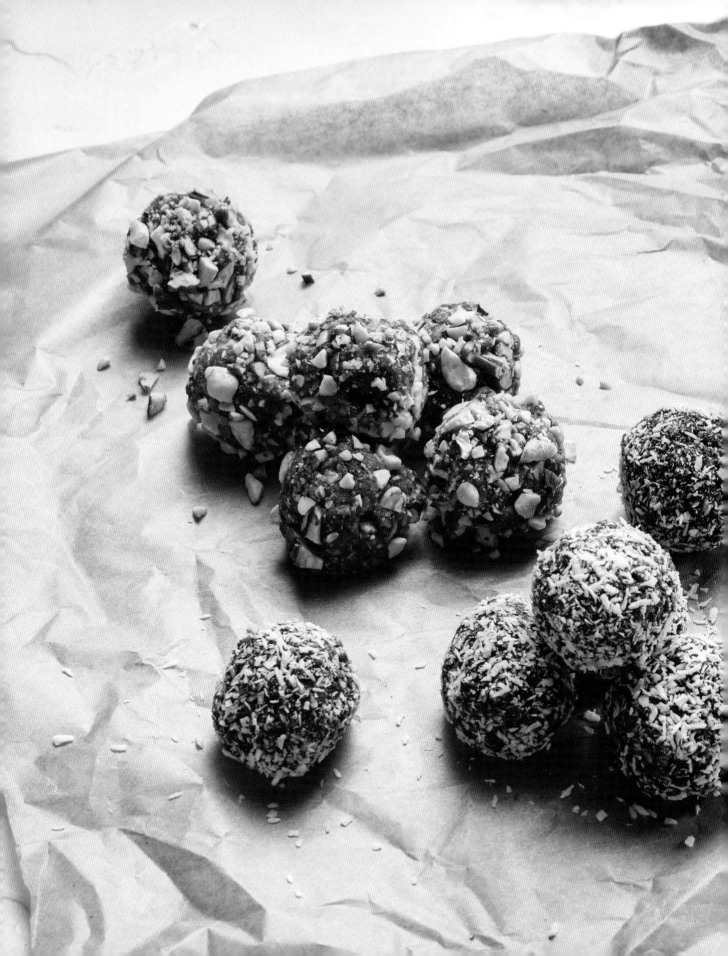

Oaty Chocolate Bliss Balls

Makes about 10 servings.

The key to making them successfully is to taste your mixture as you go.

Ingredients

1 cup gluten-free rolled oats or quinoa flakes

½ cup your favorite nut butter or sunflower seed butter

¼ cup flax seeds, freshly ground in a coffee grinder or high performance blender

2 Tbsp. unsweetened cocoa baking powder, or raw cacao powder

¼ cup raisins, soaked in ¼ cup water, then drained

2–3 Tbsp. real maple syrup (not pancake syrup), or honey

1 tsp. vanilla

1 tsp. cinnamon

Pinch of salt

1–2 Tbsp. coconut oil, melted (optional)

½ cup macaroon style shredded coconut, unsweetened

Directions

Line a baking tray with parchment paper.

Combine all ingredients, except the coconut, in a medium-sized mixing bowl. Stir dough completely. If the dough is too dry, add the optional coconut oil to moisten.

Place the shredded coconut in a small bowl. Use a spoon to scoop the dough into balls approximately 1" in size, then roll in the shredded coconut to coat your Bliss Balls completely.

Refrigerate the Bliss Balls to set. Serve chilled or room temperature.

Make Your Own Bliss Balls

Makes about 10 servings.

Modify, or create your own recipe, using this general format

Ingredients

Your favorite nut butter

Base: peanut, almond, cashew, sunflower, or tahini. Add chopped nuts (for texture): walnuts, pecans, or pistachios.

Optional extras with superfood power

Chia seeds, freshly ground flax seeds, hemp seeds, sunflower, or pumpkin seeds.

Whole food sweetener

Dates, goji berries, dried apricots, raisins, figs, or real maple syrup (not pancake syrup).

Spice up your bliss balls

Cinnamon, vanilla, lemon, nutmeg, pepper, almond extract, pumpkin pie spice, orange zest, unsweetened cocoa baking powder, or raw cacao powder.

Directions

Line a baking tray with parchment paper.

Go for a consistency that is neither too mushy, nor too dry. If the bliss balls are a little wet, that's fine. You will roll your bliss balls in a dry ingredient next, so that will take care of any stickiness issues.

Use a spoon to scoop the dough into balls approximately 1" in size. Then roll them in a chopped, dry ingredient, like chopped nuts, shredded coconut, hemp seeds, unsweetened cocoa baking powder, raw cacao powder, vanilla powder, cinnamon, cacao nibs, or protein powder.

Refrigerate the Bliss Balls to set.

Serve chilled or room temperature.

Note

Store Bliss Balls in the refrigerator for best results.

PART 2

12 Easy Do-at-Home Exercises

CONDITION YOUR BODY AND COUNTERACT HIGH BLOOD SUGAR

Exercise offers tremendous benefits for everyone, but especially for people with diabetes or other chronic illnesses. Physical exercise helps condition your muscles and lubricate your joints, which improves your mobility. In addition, doing daily physical activity, even for just 30 minutes, helps you sleep and feel better, reduces anxiety, and improves your memory. Most importantly, exercise increases blood circulation to your brain.

If you have not been in the habit of exercising, you may find it hard to start a regular routine, especially a structured one. But there is a good reason to consider starting consistent, regular exercise activity: preventing falls. Statistics show that falls are the main cause of injury, disability, and death in the elderly. It has been estimated that more than one-third of persons 65 years or older fall each year, due to any number of causes, from simple tripping on the sidewalk to slipping in the bathtub or shower. But you can also experience falls due to the improper working of the balancing mechanism located in the inner ear, or impairment of your vision or depth perception, due to some type of limitation of your brain's signal processing mechanism or due to medication side effects.

The best way to decrease the chance of falling is to maintain as normal a balance and gait as possible. This requires good muscle tone, comfortable joint motion, and awareness of your surroundings. To achieve those, you need proper nerve function along with adequate concentration; these are necessary to make movement adjustments based on continuous input from your inner ears (where one's sense of equilibrium comes from) regarding your body in motion. You also need good vision that provides awareness of your surroundings.

The exercises I am suggesting are designed to be practiced in place and do not involve walking around. Rather than increasing the possibility of a fall, as you may be concerned about, these exercises will go a long way to preventing one.

The Benefits of Exercise

Before you peruse or begin trying the exercises, take some time now to read the following sections on the many benefits of regular exercise. These include improving your general well-being, muscle stability, joint mobility, and even your brain function. In addition, I will discuss the benefits regarding heart health and lung conditioning. Furthermore, according to the CDC, among adults aged 45 to 64 in the United states, 44% have prediabetes or diabetes, so I also point out how exercise can help lower blood sugar, though you cannot expect exercise alone to prevent the progression of prediabetes to Type 2 diabetes! That requires altering your diet, which is the goal of the recipes in this book.

General well-being

It is known that physical activity can help you sleep better and feel better. It can reduce the risk of twenty chronic health conditions, including heart disease and some cancers.

Exercise, in this context, is defined as any activity done to maintain and improve physical health and mental well-being. You can exercise outdoors or indoors. Outdoor exercises include walking, running, cycling, swimming, rowing, hiking, or playing sports; indoor exercises include dancing, weight or interval training, or skipping rope. There are many choices! Clearly, some of these can be done either outside or inside, either alone or in the company of others. Dynamic exercises such as running can improve your blood circulation, whereas static exercises such as weightlifting can increase your muscle strength as well as your blood pressure.

While the type of exercise can be tailored based on your goal and age, doing any exercise is better than doing none. In fact, the psychological and physiological benefits of adhering to an exercise routine are more pronounced when you recognize the value of exercise and voluntarily embrace it.[1] Daily exercise lasting at least 30 minutes has been shown to reduce anxiety and improve memory.

It has been clearly demonstrated that persons who remain sedentary have a higher risk of cardiovascular disease, such as heart attack and stroke, compared to those who exercise and expend at least 700 kcal (calories) of energy per week. According to the US Centers for Disease Control and Prevention, people who are physically active for about 150 minutes a week have a 33% lower risk of dying from all causes than those who are physically inactive.[2] This means that by exercising about 30 minutes each day of the week, you can significantly cut your risk of dying prematurely.

A recent study showed that for every 2,000 steps you take each day, your risk for premature death may fall by 8 to 11 percent.[3]

Muscle stability

As we get older, metabolic activities inside each cell in the body produce agents known as "Reactive Oxygen Species" (ROS) that can cause damage to proteins and/or genes.

1. Kennedy AB, Resnick PB (May 2015). "Mindfulness and Physical Activity". *American Journal of Lifestyle Medicine.* 9 (3): 3221–3323. doi:10.1177/1559827614564546. S2CID 73116017.

2. cdc.gov/physicalactivity/basics/pa-health/index.htm

3. Prospective Associations of Daily Step Counts and Intensity With Cancer and Cardiovascular Disease Incidence and Mortality and All-Cause Mortality. Borja del Pozo Cruz, PhD1; Matthew N. Ahmadi, PhD2; I-Min Lee, MBBS, ScD3,4; et al. *JAMA Intern Med.* Published online September 12, 2022. doi:10.1001/jamainternmed.2022.4000

For example, the atrophy of skeletal muscles that causes them to perform less efficiently is thought to be due to increased production of ROS. Regular muscle activity keeps the metabolic pathways working efficiently while reducing the production of ROS.

The importance of muscle function becomes clear when you consider a potentially life-threatening situation that necessitates your immediate movement, such as jumping out of the way of a car or walking through a crowd. With conditioned muscles that work with more efficiency than unconditioned ones, you can react and move faster.

To clearly understand the concept of muscle conditioning, it helps to know something about muscles in general and how they function in particular. A skeletal muscle contains multiple bundles composed of three different types of fibers, each based on distinct metabolic, contractile, and motor unit properties. The primary function of muscle is contraction. When a muscle contracts, the fibers release signaling molecules believed to be responsible for the health benefits of exercise. Another major contribution from muscle function is maintaining your body's stable internal temperature. During metabolic activities needed to produce ATP—the fuel that cells need to perform their internal operations—a lot of potential energy is lost as heat. In this process, every cell contributes to body heat, but the metabolic activity of muscles is responsible for 85% of it. You can see the critical part muscles play in providing heat when you shiver in extreme cold, as your muscles are attempting to generate heat.

Aerobic exercises of long duration such as running, swimming, and dancing require a steady supply of oxygen to generate ATP within cells. Anaerobic exercises such as sprinting and weightlifting are usually of shorter duration, during which ATP is produced through the breakdown of glucose without using much oxygen. Although glucose gives you a sudden spurt of energy, it can also result in the formation of lactic acid, which, when accumulated inside muscle fibers, can inhibit the ATP formation that you need for longer duration exercise. However, muscle conditioning can mitigate this by building more blood vessels to drain the acid. Most common exercises are partially aerobic and anaerobic.

Muscle strength comes from your muscle size, the strength of the nerve signals reaching the muscle, and mechanical factors such as joint capabilities, as well as the training you do to build muscle size. Although the number of muscle fibers cannot be increased through exercise, muscle can grow larger by adding new protein filaments alongside existing muscle cells. However, this may prove to be difficult to maintain as one gets older. In fact, muscle strength and the stamina for sustained physical activities both decline with age, largely due to the reduction in hormone levels and accumulation of damages to genes.

Joint mobility

The human skeleton, composed of 270 bones at birth, is the internal scaffolding that makes it possible for a person to stand, sit, and move around on two feet. The bones are composed mostly of calcium minerals and reach their maximum density around age 21. Your bones are about 14% of your total body weight.

Where two bones meet, a joint is created that connects the bones into a functional unit that allows for different types and degrees of movement. Some joints—such as knee, elbow, and shoulder—are self-lubricating. But injury, infection, surgery, or prolonged nonuse can result in a condition called fibrosis that limits the joint lubrication and thus the joint's function. Now you can understand the importance of regular exercise in maintaining joint functionality and the physical capability of the body.

Brain function

Each behavior you have consists of an input that triggers it, then nerve impulses that go through the brain to process it, and finally an output that manifests itself in your actions. Doing physical exercise follows the same general principle of input, processing, and output. Exercise thus helps keep your brain functioning, which can add to your alertness as you age.

One evidence of the importance of exercise for the brain is the finding that declining mental functions are almost twice as common among adults who are inactive as those who are active.[4]

In addition, people with high blood sugar had more than twice the risk of developing dementia than those without it. Persistent elevation of blood glucose could lead to glucose attaching to proteins and thus creating "advanced glycation end products" that are thought to be responsible for interfering with brain functions.[5] This means that if you are diabetic, physical activity is one of the best means of preventing deterioration of your brain function.

Ideally, most adults should get at least 150 minutes of moderate intensity physical activity on a weekly basis. This does not mean that the activity has to be uninterrupted. It can be broken into smaller segments such as 30 minutes a day. Even a simple exercise such as walking between 3,800 and 9,800 steps each day can reduce your risk of mental decline.[6]

---

4. Cross-sectional association between physical activity level and subjective cognitive decline among US adults aged ≥45 years. 2015 Preventive Medicine, Volume 141, December 2020, 106279 John D. Omura, David R. Brown, Lisa C. McGuire, et al.

5. Aragno, M.; Mastrocola, R. Dietary sugars and endogenous formation of advanced glycation end products: Emerging mechanisms of disease. *Nutrients* 2017, *9*, 385.

6. Association of Daily Step Count and Intensity With Incident Dementia in 78,430 Adults Living in the UK. Borja del Pozo Cruz, PhD1; Matthew Ahmadi, PhD2; Sharon L. Naismith, PhD3; et al. *JAMA Neurol.* Published online September 6, 2022. doi:10.1001/jamaneurol.2022.2672

Blood sugar control

Muscles can use either glucose or fatty acids as their fuel to produce the energy needed for exercising. Based on the type of meal you eat and how digestible the food components are that you consume, your blood sugar levels will start spiking about 60 to 90 minutes after eating. This corresponds with the release of insulin from the pancreas, which informs cells of the presence of glucose outside the cell wall.

The gene in charge of glucose acquisition then activates "transporters" that move to the cell wall to pick up the glucose molecules outside and bring them in. However, the quantity of insulin released matches the level of the spike in blood glucose only up to a point. This could be due to the presence of fatty acids in the bloodstream, which inform the pancreas about the availability of an alternative fuel, cutting the further release of insulin.

Your skeletal muscles burn roughly 90 mg of glucose each minute during continuous physical activity. This is to be expected because physical activity dominates the body's use of energy. Therefore, exercising immediately after a meal provides glucose from carbohydrates in the meal and insulin released from the pancreas that aids muscle glucose uptake. In addition, a muscle warmed by exercise has been found to activate transporters that can bring in more glucose even when insulin is not present outside. In short, people with diabetes can benefit by just taking a walk right after a meal. However, for exercise to be of practical use in controlling blood sugar one has to be prepared to exercise after every carbohydrate-containing meal, as well as able to adjust the duration of exercise corresponding to the carbohydrate intake. I submit that both of these are not practical in daily life.

Even just standing up for a few minutes throughout the day and after meals can lower blood glucose on average by 9.5%. However, the best option is to walk two to five minutes every 30 minutes throughout the day, which will result in better glucose control. Keep in mind, however, you might develop an increased appetite following exercise, which could offset your attempt at glucose control.[7]

The most effective exercise, however, is between meals, even though your blood insulin level is at its lowest. In these situations, cellular energy production is influenced by three other hormones: glucagon, epinephrine, and growth hormone. When you exercise, your muscles send a message to the brain requesting additional fuel. The brain, in turn, sends signals to cause the release of these additional hormones. Glucagon stimulates the release of stored glucose from the liver, while epinephrine and growth hormone stimulate the release of fatty

---

7. The Acute Effects of Interrupting Prolonged Sitting Time in Adults with Standing and Light-Intensity Walking on Biomarkers of Cardiometabolic Health in Adults: A Systematic Review and Meta-analysis. Aidan J. Buffey, Matthew P. Herring, Christina K. Langley, et al. *Sports Medicine* 52:1765–1787 (February 2022)

acids from fat cells. The release of glucose from the liver helps maintain your blood glucose level so that nerves in the brain can function, while muscles rely on the fatty acids for their energy production. The use of released fatty acids from fat cells is why exercise can help you lose weight, albeit very small amounts are lost during an exercise routine.

But note that this metabolic fact means that in the long term, the availability of fatty acids ultimately determines the level of blood sugar control you can achieve from exercise. As you get older, and you are unable to maintain the same level of physical activity, you tend to gain weight from fat cells while losing muscle fiber from reduced exercise.

Heart health

The heart is a four-chambered pump made of muscle. It is responsible for sending blood to all parts of the body. The left ventricle sends blood carrying nutrients and oxygen to every cell in the body. The aorta is the main vessel that carries blood from the left ventricle. Branches of the aorta—the arteries—supply blood to every part of the body. Arteries further subdivide into smaller blood vessels called capillaries. Along the capillary walls are perforations, or tiny holes, that allow the fluid part of blood carrying nutrients—but not the red blood cells—to leak into the outside and reach nearby cells. (However, red cells can get out when there is injury to the capillary wall, causing bleeding. White blood cells can also get out when openings are created in the capillary wall by enzymes released during inflammation.)

The fluid leaking out from the blood allows each cell to pick up needed nutrients, as cells absorb whichever nutrients they need based on their functional specialization. In turn, cells discharge waste and carbon dioxide into blood carried by veins to return to the right side of the heart. Veins empty the blood into the right ventricle, which pumps the blood to the lungs where carbon dioxide is released into the air and oxygen is picked up. The oxygenated blood returns to the left side of the heart to repeat the cycle.

Regular exercise provides two benefits for the heart. On the one hand, it improves the supply of oxygen and nutrients, which increases the efficiency of the heart muscle. On the other hand, it conditions your heart muscle, which can then pump more blood with less effort compared to an unconditioned heart. In other words, systematic use of the heart makes heart muscles more efficient in their pumping performance. This means that you can have a lower number of heart beats in the long run, which can prolong the life of your heart muscle.

Lung conditioning

Every human being has to overcome an unavoidable challenge to survive on the earth: adapting to living in an environment of air, not water as it did in the womb. Before birth, a baby is surrounded by water, protected from the elements, and getting nourishment and oxygen fed through the umbilical cord. It is lulled into a state of meditation by the rhythmic beat of the mother's heart. Then at some moment, it is suddenly thrust into the unfamiliar medium of air and forced to acquire oxygen and nutrients by itself.

Taking a breath is the first act the baby performs, and the difficulty of that is evidenced in the cry heard during inhalation and exhalation of its first breath of air through the mouth. The air moving through the bronchial tubes displaces the water that until now has been keeping the air sacs at the end of the breathing tubes filled. From that first breath onward, the air sacs are meant to be kept open so that carbon dioxide produced during metabolic activities in the body can be exchanged for oxygen from the outside air.

Considering the importance of oxygen to life, nature made breathing to be automatic, though there is also some fine tuning of it in the control centers located in the brain. Based on the need for oxygen during different metabolic activities, the brain can increase the number of breaths per minute, such as during physical exercise. Movement of air into the lungs is accomplished by the action of muscles that expand the chest cavity, while moving air out is independent of skeletal muscle contraction, as it is accomplished by the contraction of fibers lining the air sacs that were stretched by the air during inhalation.

It is well known that for breathing to be effective, air passages have to be open; so the structural integrity of air sacs must thus be maintained. Chronic inflammation of the air sacs—such as that from smoking, inhalation of asbestos particles, and infections from bacteria and fungi—can impede air flow and the oxygenation of blood, either by narrowing the air passages or by reducing the efficiency of the exchange of air in the air sacs.

Here is a simple exercise that can improve the conditioning of chest wall muscles and that of the fibers of the air sacs. Try this exercise to strengthen the muscles involved in air movement.

Simple Deep Breathing Exercise

1. Sit comfortably with your legs firmly planted.

2. Take a deep breath to a mental count of four.

3. Hold the breath for a mental count of five.

4. Purse your lips and force the air through the lips to a mental count of twenty or more.

Repeat this exercise as many times as you are comfortable and as often as time permits. See below for another exercise routine using deep breathing that can also help you condition the fibers lining the air sacs.

Instructions for the Easy Exercises

Here are 12 different exercises, and each has an accompanying animated video showing you how to do it. You can access the videos by clicking the QR code next to the exercise title. These exercises are easy to execute in the comfort of your home, at any time you feel the desire, to offset boredom or anxiety or simply put, when you have nothing else to do.

Note that you don't have to do all of them, or in the same sequence presented. However, I urge you to do one or more of these exercises whenever you get some free time. Some of them can be done anywhere and anytime. For example, when you are bored or when you are just sitting around on the couch, do the deep breathing exercise, paying attention to the movement of air through your nose and that of your chest wall muscles. Similarly, you can do the breathing exercise when you are listening to something on TV or during commercials, or when you are waiting for service in a restaurant or any other similar situation.

Toe taps are an excellent activity when you are a passenger in a car, train, or airplane, or when there is a dull moment while you are sitting, watching a stage event or sport, during a meeting or while waiting for an appointment. You could also do toe taps in the standing position when you are forced to stand in a train, subway, slow moving commuter vehicle, using one leg after another.

You can do the leg-related exercises every morning before you get out of your bed. In fact, every time you lie down, you have an opportunity to do one or more of the leg exercises. If you have a history of feeling dizzy when you stand up suddenly after being on your back for some time, this could be due to a condition called postural hypotension. Doing leg exercises before getting up to a sitting position or doing toe tapping in the sitting position before standing up, could speed delivery of blood to your brain and limit the degree of dizziness from postural hypotension.

Over time, you may find other opportunities to put into practice these exercises. You may even want to invent new exercises based on these that you enjoy doing to keep your muscles, joints, and lungs functionally efficient.

Note: You should first get your doctor's or physical therapist's advice as to what types of exercises you can comfortably do. For example, if you are already out of shape and not yet limber, you may not be able to perform some of these exercises, especially those involving bending your back. Make sure the sofa or bed you use is strong enough to support you.

1. Dynamic arms sweep. To perform this exercise, stand upright with your feet hip-width apart resting comfortably on the ground. Sweep both hands to the left in the horizontal plane, keeping your elbows straight. Have your left palm facing forward, and your right palm facing upward. Gradually move both arms to the right, then back to the left. Increase the number of repetitions as you get more comfortable with the exercise.

2. Dynamic front arms. To perform this exercise, stand upright with your feet resting hip-width apart comfortably on the ground. While taking a deep breath, spread your arms to their respective sides, with elbows straight and palms facing forward. While exhaling, gradually move both arms to meet the palms in front of you. Open the arms again to the sides. Repeat the exercise at least three times. Increase the number of repetitions as you get more comfortable with the exercise.

3. Dynamic top arms. To perform this exercise, stand upright with your feet resting hip-width apart comfortably on the ground. Spread your arms to their respective sides in the horizontal plane with elbows straight and palms facing upward. Gradually move both arms to meet palms above your head. Open the arms again and repeat the exercise at least three times. Increase the number of repetitions as you get more comfortable with the exercise.

4. Deep breathing exercise. To perform this exercise, sit on a sofa or the bedside, with your feet resting comfortably on the ground. Rest your hands on your thighs, palms facing upwards. Bend your fingers so that the thumb touches the tip of your index (pointer) finger. Holding that position, take a deep breath through your nose to a silent count of four. Hold your breath to a silent count of five. Exhale through your nose to a silent count of six. Then hold your breath and relax to a silent count of seven. Repeat the exercise three more times, with the thumb touching each of the other three fingers in sequence.

5. Shoulder stretch. To perform this exercise, sit upright on a sofa or bedside with your legs resting comfortably on the ground. Keep your hands with palms together in front of your legs. Bend your head gently as far down as you can with your fingers pointing down. Then, keeping one hand pointing down as far as you can go, lift and move the other hand up over your head as far back as possible to stretch your shoulder. Gently reverse the movement to bring your hand back down to the floor as much as possible. Repeat the exercise using the other hand, then repeat stretching with both hands together over the head. Repeat the whole routine at least three times. Increase the number of repetitions as you get more comfortable with the exercise,

 **6. Toe taps.** To perform this exercise, sit on a sofa or bedside with your feet resting comfortably on the ground. You may use any comfortable footwear or be barefoot. Lift the right leg a few inches, point your toes down, and swing your foot backwards. Tap your toes as you move your foot forwards until you can go no further. Then tap back to the starting position and put your heel down. Then do the exercise with your left foot. Repeat the exercise three times and increase the number of repetitions as you get more comfortable with the exercise.

 **7. Deadbugs.** To perform this exercise, lie flat on your back on the floor, or on a sofa or bed, with your palms facing down at your side. If necessary, you may use a pillow under your knees. Bend one knee upwards, then stretch the leg back down. Repeat the process using the other leg. Then, repeat the same activity with both knees bent at the same time, using your hands to gently pull your knees down towards your stomach. Repeat the exercise at least three times. Increase the number of repetitions as you get more comfortable with the exercise.

 **8. V-ups.** To perform this exercise, lie flat on your back on the floor, or on a sofa or bed, with your palms facing down at your side. Lift your head up and extend your hands over your legs to get your fingertips towards your toes as far as you can go. You may bend your knee as you stretch your hands forward. Immediately lay your head back down while bringing your arms back. Repeat the exercise at least three times. Increase the number of repetitions as you get more comfortable with the exercise.

 **9. Leg lift.** To perform this exercise, lie flat on your back on the floor, or on a sofa or bed, with your palms facing down.

Lift one leg from your hip in the fully extended position without bending the knee by a few inches and immediately put it down. Repeat the same with the other leg. Then lift both legs up together in the fully extended position by a few inches. Immediately bring the legs down together. Repeat the exercise at least three times. Increase the number of repetitions as you get more comfortable with the exercise.

10. Shoulder stand. You should be careful when doing this exercise; otherwise you could hurt your back. To perform this exercise, lie flat on your back on the floor, or on a sofa or bed, with your palms facing down. Lift both legs up together in the fully extended position, bending at your hip joint while keeping your knees straight. Lift your hips up and support your back with your palms to help keep your legs as vertical as possible. Your body will be almost in an L-shape. Hold that position to a mental count of ten. Increase the duration of holding your legs up as you get more comfortable with the exercise.

11. Air cycle. To perform this exercise, lie flat on your back on the floor, or on a sofa or bed, with your palms facing down at your side. Lift both legs up together in the fully extended position, bending at your hip joint while keeping your knees straight. Lift your hips up and support your back with your palms to help keep your legs as vertical as possible. Your body will be almost in an L-shape. While holding that position, move your feet and legs as if you were bicycling to a mental count of ten. Increase the duration of air cycling as you get more comfortable with the exercise.

12. Leg flip. To perform this exercise, lie flat on your back on the floor, or on a sofa or bed. Lift both legs up together in the fully extended position, bending at your hip joint while keeping your knees straight. Lift your hips up, supporting your back with your palms if needed. Keep moving your legs as far back as possible, bringing your toes over your head. Your body will be almost in a U-shape. Reverse the movement slowly until your heels are back on the sofa. Repeat the exercise at least three times. Increase the number of repetitions as you get more comfortable with the exercise.

PART 3

How to Stay Motivated

CONTROL YOUR WEIGHT AND YOUR DIABETES

It would be natural for you to allow your fear of yet another failure to hold you back from adopting new eating and exercise habits. But as long as your intention is clear and precise, it can help you follow your chosen path to your goal. Go over the plan in your mind periodically and visualize how you can overcome the difficulties in front of you. Do not allow yourself to be discouraged by one day of overeating or going off your promise to eat healthy foods.

The more you discover your inner strength, the more confident you will become. Remind yourself that before you were diagnosed with Type 2 diabetes, you lived, perhaps for many decades, having normal blood sugar levels. It was not a change in your genetic makeup that made you diabetic during your midlife but a change in your lifestyle. And that is something that is completely within your control.

To help you keep your motivation to establish a new lifestyle related to modifying your diet and exercise habits, let me suggest the following five steps. But keep in mind that your motivation becomes real only when it comes from within you.

STEP 1. Believe in yourself

You have the power to modify your diet-related behaviors to achieve proper blood sugar control and your exercise habits to keep your joints lubricated. What I would like you to be clear on is the fact that the dietary changes I suggest in this book are going to change your metabolism at the cellular level. By repeating the new way of eating at every meal, every day, you will gradually shift away from being a patient with Type 2 diabetes to an independent person confident in your ability to control your blood sugar on your own.

First you have to be willing to look for your inner strength—and more importantly, to believe in it. The most significant motivating factor, the one that drove you to seek medical treatment of diabetes, is that of survival. In this book I offer you an improved quality of life—the joy of not just surviving but thriving—as the incentive to use dietary changes rather than medications to control your blood sugar.

I would also add that although your primary assignment is to keep your blood sugar under control using dietary adjustments, there is more to life than simply being free of diabetes. Daily exercise, as explained in this book, along with other physical and mental activities, is the means to achieve that. That is why this book covers both diet and exercise as complementary prescriptions to help you live healthy for longer.

As your brain adjusts to your new way of eating, you will become aware that the old way of eating still reappears from time to time, based on overconsumption that makes you feel full. This is to be expected because you have been practicing that way of eating for years, if not decades. It could take up to six months of repetition for your brain to establish the new way of eating as your default mechanism.

The surest way to make this happen is to understand that all your actions start with a thought process. It is understandable that you consider thoughts already embedded into your psyche to be both real, irrefutable, and easily executable. But be confident in the steps you are taking based on what you have learned in this book. Start each day believing in your ability to fulfill your expectation of controlling your blood sugar through your own actions. As you change your thoughts, you will begin to change your habits.

Once you start seeing a lowering of your blood glucose level, however small the drop may be, you will begin appreciating and respecting the dietary changes that made it possible. Keep in mind that small victories are the building blocks to creating the strong willpower you need to succeed. Slowly, you will develop a deeper trust in yourself—the mark of self-confidence. This self-confidence will then lead you into more victories, and thus you will build a self-sustaining motivational tool. Now is the time to plan for the rest of your diabetes-free life.

STEP 2. Concentrate more on the rewards than on the difficulties

When it comes to implementing dietary changes, you will run into a stumbling block as you seek not to inconvenience others, especially your immediate family members and close friends. You will find yourself making excuses. The fact is, such attitudes you expressed in the past may have enabled others to brainwash you into believing they agree with you. They may even have expressed their own explanations to make you believe that they are supporting you, creating an inescapable circular belief system.

To escape this trap, concentrate on your own rewards: preserving your kidney function, protecting your vision, keeping your limbs intact, supporting your heart function, being able to think clearly, and enjoying the company of others. The key is to assume personal responsibility for your physical health, and that includes maintaining your blood sugar control. Every time you concentrate on your own rewards, you increase your self-confidence to continue on the path to a healthy life.

STEP 3. Live in the present and plan for a better future

Almost everyone trusts information that comes from a reliable source, such as the family physician. Ideally, patients want to leave the doctor's office with an optimistic attitude or at least with assurance that the medical expert is up-to-date on the information regarding your condition and will do everything they can to correct the perceived problem.

You may feel that I am asking you to go against what you believed until now to be the only way to control blood sugar. However, in reality, what I am asking you to do is to apply what is called "Occam's razor," the term used to abandon unnecessarily convoluted scientific theories such as the insulin resistance theory. Occam's razor pleads for "shaving away" complicated illogical assumptions to reach a simpler, more logical explanation about a scientific conundrum, in this case the cause of Type 2 diabetes. According to Occam's razor, most often the simplest explanation is the correct one.

In addition, recognize that I am not selling any medical treatments, supplements, or gadgets to control your blood sugar. I am not roping you into months of subscribing to anything. My only goal has been that you read this book and absorb the knowledge I have been sharing so that you can make the simple dietary changes needed to control your blood sugar on your own.

Remember that the former dietary lifestyle you had leads to the potential of more than a 50% chance of suffering significant complications from diabetes, as well as significant side effects from treatments. With confidence, embrace the new knowledge you learned from this book. Embark on putting what you have learned into practice, supported by scientific evidence, and prepare for a future devoid of anxiety related to blood sugar level fluctuations, developing the serious complications of diabetes, or suffering the side effects of diabetic medications.

STEP 4. Remain vigilant

It is likely that you will get advice from others regarding how to accomplish blood sugar control. While some of it may be based on their own personal experiences, others may be anecdotal based solely on what they heard or read. As a social being, your sincerity and emotional need to be agreeable may compel you to believe in some truth in what they are telling you. You can be courteous and thank them, but be vigilant and critical; analyze the information, after checking their sources and evidence. There are many non-scientific, if not outright fraudulent, claims and treatments being marketed for Type 2 diabetes, so be selective in your follow-up scrutiny. Otherwise, you may be sold a false path to health, or a completely bogus product—one that will have no real impact on your ability to control your blood sugar.

Your biggest challenge is going to come from healthcare practitioners who believe that glucose control is synonymous with diabetes control. Compounding this are the stresses and worries of daily living. Medical practitioners will try to persuade you to keep taking at least some medication along with your dietary changes. They may tell you about others who have achieved blood sugar control using medications. If you come across something logical, use your own intuition to determine its usefulness.

STEP 5. Be an inspiration for others

Soon after you start on your path to a healthier diet, you may become aware that others are noticing your effort to change. Some may find it hard to understand what you are doing and insist that you follow your doctor's advice. They may criticize your naïveté in believing that there is a natural way to control Type 2 diabetes. They will say "it's in the family" and imply that you cannot avoid it. However, after this initial disapproval, when they realize how serious you are, you will be surprised to see they will likely help you by accommodating your dietary changes. Those with Type 2 diabetes may even try to follow your efforts, especially if they have been afraid to change their dietary habits because of unknown consequences. Your success can become their source of inspiration when they see an ordinary person living a healthy life using simple dietary changes.

You don't need to tell or advertise to others what you are doing—unless you want to. Even if your example gives hope to only one person diagnosed with high blood sugar, you can be proud of saving that person from lifelong anxiety and potential complications related to Type 2 diabetes. Keep in mind that most people are taking medications for diabetes under the mindset that medication is the best and only way to go. This mindset has been created and deeply entrenched by the repeated assurances of the medical community about the need for medication to control blood sugar level. This is reinforced on TV, in pharmacies and supermarkets, and in advertising on the internet and in magazines. It is going to take time and persistence to change this rigid mentality. But it all starts with an example—you!

One way to share your inspiration is by forming a network of people trying to accomplish the same objective. Share the pleasure of the dietary changes you have experienced and help others feel that you are as enthusiastic to see them succeed as you are about your own success. This reinforces each individual's determination through the sharing of your commitment to overcome resistance. In fact, this is the best way to discover your own weaknesses and solidify your own determination. In the end, you will find that others, like you, feel stronger when meeting people who have learned from past unhealthy habits and have ultimately changed them.

EPILOGUE

I have two objectives in writing this book. The first is to help YOU learn how to reduce the total food energy you consume by concentrating on the enjoyment of eating. Nature gives us a clue by putting all the nutrients an adult body needs into natural packages: vegetables, fruits, nuts, and other edibles that require chewing. The more you chew, the more percentage of a bite of food you enjoy; additionally, your own control centers inform you when to stop eating that food by reducing the intensity of enjoyment.

My second objective is to help you control your blood sugar level by reducing your intake of glucose. For this you have to voluntarily reduce the amount of grain-based foods to one-half of what you presently consume, or at least no more than 25% to 30% of your daily consumption of calories.

My explanation is logical, clear, and makes more sense than the concept of insulin resistance. To review, we know that most cells, muscle cells in particular, derive more energy using fatty acid than glucose—similar to a hybrid car sometimes using electricity rather than gasoline to produce energy. Given that, it is easy to imagine that the presence of fatty acid in the blood from a diet rich in complex carbohydrates will cause muscle cells to burn those fatty acids rather than glucose. From that, it is easy to imagine how the unburned glucose remains in the bloodstream, leading to high blood sugar, leading to a diagnosis of Type 2 diabetes. This explanation clarifies why dietary change to reduce the formation of fatty acids in the body forces cells such as muscles to use more glucose, as they are designed to do, to control blood sugar.

I have stated in this book what I believe to be the scientific truth. I am well aware of the fact that "truth" is what a person is willing to believe, regardless of facts that may suggest otherwise. This means that while we may not be able to alter the perception of truth in anyone not willing to entertain new information, we can defend facts with objective evidence. I ask you to step back from any emotional loyalty you may have to your healthcare provider and activate your intellectual curiosity regarding the reason for developing Type 2 diabetes.

Let me be clear. I am not disputing the evidence gathered by experts in diabetes, only the interpretations of that evidence. For example, my theory uses the normal role of fatty acids as fuel for metabolic activities at the cellular level to explain the elevation of blood glucose and

Type 2 diabetes. Mine is a different interpretation than that of diabetologists who interpret the same evidence as a sign of cellular "resistance" to insulin. While the diabetologists justify the use of medications, including the insulin you are supposedly resistant to, to overcome cellular resistance, my interpretation does not even need the concept of insulin resistance to explain blood glucose elevation in a patient with Type 2 diabetes. In fact, my explanation justifies that only diet modification is needed for the management of Type 2 diabetes.

However, be warned that the contemporary media have made it easy to propagate "alternate facts." My response to that is best summarized by a great statement from the senator from New York, Daniel Patrick Moynihan: "Everyone is entitled to their own opinion, but not to their own facts." In other words, diabetes experts can interpret laboratory findings and clinical evidence to fit their beliefs, but they can't escape the facts.

Therefore, my position is: *Be firm, be impartial, be confident, be truthful, be persistent.*

Let me conclude by pointing out the differences to control blood sugar level in Type 2 diabetes that I am proposing in this book compared to the conventional paradigm. The practice guidelines currently used are based on a three-pronged approach: diet, exercise, and drugs. On the surface, what I am proposing in this book may appear to be the same. However, there are important differences.

Let me start in reverse order with the drugs, especially insulin and medications that force insulin release from the pancreas. The codification of insulin treatment for controlling Type 2 diabetes looks normal when viewed through the lens of a treatment paradigm for Type 1 diabetes. In Type 1 diabetes, normalizing blood sugar can be used to determine the dose of insulin because the primary defect here is an inability to utilize glucose in the bloodstream due to non-availability of insulin. However, in Type 2 diabetes, the problem is an oversupply of glucose, primarily coming from grains and grain-based foods, a completely different causative factor.

Yet endocrinologists explain the elevation of blood sugar as the manifestation of "insulin resistance," without offering any scientific proof. It is for this reason that I do not recommend routine use of insulin for the management of Type 2 diabetes, unless endocrinologists can show proof that insulin treatment lowers the incidence of long-term diabetic complications.

As for exercise, I am all for it; but not for guaranteed control of blood sugar. I promote exercise as a way to condition the body for greater general health. Although exercise may work for some people in the early stages of Type 2 diabetes to burn glucose and lower their blood sugar, this degree of glucose reduction cannot be sustained by exercise alone, due to aging-related loss of muscle strength. As you get older, you simply do not burn as much glucose when exercising.

As for diet modification, I believe whole-heartedly with the need to lower the intake of one's total food energy (calories). But the approach I am presenting in this book is to remove the root cause of excess glucose supply in the present day diet rather than promoting the use of drugs and exercise to move it out of the blood. In this regard, we have given you numerous delicious and easy-to-make recipes to follow. You are free to continue to enjoy food preparation using vegetables and animal products as you have done before. The only condition I suggest is to select dishes that require chewing; that is how you can modify how you eat from meal choices based on consumption to those based on enjoyment, until this new way of eating becomes automatic. This important lifestyle modification along with exercise then becomes the foundation of an active diabetes-free life.

Let me be clear. In writing this book, I am not trying to point an accusing finger at diabetes experts who were taught the conceptual basis of diabetes management by their professors who themselves believed in it. Like any new scientific theory, it takes hold and lasts until someone is able to burst the bubble of a false theory by introducing a more logical and provable theory. I suggest that this can be achieved by compelling the proponents of the current theory of the cause of Type 2 diabetes to explain and defend it through evidence beyond reasonable doubt of the insulin resistance theory.

To accomplish that, I invite you to ask your doctor the following questions:

1. How do oral medications reduce the glucose in my blood?

2. What is the reason for my body to resist insulin and not other hormones?

3. Is there a test to know the degree of my insulin resistance?

4. My friend needs dialysis in spite of taking insulin. Will I have to do the same?

5. Why do so many diabetics end up with severe consequences if they were taking medications or injecting insulin?

6. Will my children develop diabetes? Have scientists discovered a gene for diabetes?

I am convinced that the rather vague answers you get will prove to you the greater logic and reliability of my dietary recommendations to control Type 2 diabetes.

APPENDIX: DR. JOHN'S ANSWERS TO FREQUENTLY ASKED QUESTIONS

What is the difference between Type 1 and Type 2 diabetes?

There are two common forms of diabetes, Type 1 and Type 2.

Type 1 diabetes. In this form of diabetes, the special cells in the pancreas that are responsible for producing insulin do not function adequately. Insulin is the hormone messenger that tells the body's cells to allow glucose from the bloodstream into them. The cells use glucose to produce the energy they need for their normal functions.

In general, Type 1 diabetes occurs when people develop a non-functioning pancreas. Without glucose, cells starve in vital organs, leading to death. In most cases, Type 1 diabetes occurs in infancy, although it can also occur years after birth. Type 1 diabetes is a real hormonal disease.

It was established that Type 1 diabetic patients need insulin, due to their lack of natural production of insulin. This did not occur until the 1920s, when a group of Canadian researchers isolated and purified insulin that could be used to treat Type 1 diabetes. Prior to that, a person with Type 1 diabetes did not live long following the onset of the disease.

Type 2 diabetes. In this form of diabetes, it is believed that the pancreas produces insulin but three types of cells in the body—muscle, liver, and fat cells—do not respond to it. This leaves the glucose in the bloodstream, resulting in high blood sugar.

The evolution of the above concept explaining Type 2 diabetes is worth understanding because the explanation does not appear to be correct. Originally, it was thought that high blood sugar in adults was similar to that in children, i.e., a lack of insulin production by the pancreas. Thus, it was originally called "adult onset diabetes." However, when it was found that adults with elevated glucose levels had plenty of insulin, the terminology was changed to "non-insulin-dependent diabetes," as medical science did not understand the reason for the high blood sugar. Eventually, around the 1930s, a test was created where patients were injected with insulin and were still found to have high blood sugar. This led to a theory that body cells must be "resistant" to the insulin. This hypothesis became commonly known as "insulin resistance."

Oddly enough, medical science has not yet been able to explain why this supposed insulin resistance occurs, nor by exactly what biological mechanism it happens. It remains unexplained why billions of cells suddenly switch to resist the presence of insulin to allow glucose to enter them when those cells didn't have the problem before. One of the most suspicious (and biologically illogical) elements of this theory is that insulin resistance does not occur in all the body's cells. There are 200 types of cells in the body, but the theory states that insulin resistance occurs in only three main groups of cells: 1) muscle cells that have not been warmed up (inactive muscle cells), 2) the liver, and 3) fat cells. No matter how much biological science you know or don't know, it is clear this theory does not make sense. Why would only three types of cells become resistant to insulin?

In addition, there is no finding of any agents that block insulin nor any proof of cellular changes. No research has discovered or demonstrated an actual agent that blocks the binding of insulin with the insulin receptor on cells at the time Type 2 diabetes is diagnosed. In contrast, with many diseases, an agent such as an antibody has been found to block the utilization of molecules in cells. Similarly, there is no proof of any type of change in cells that might make them suddenly resist insulin. Research has not identified any differences in cells that are supposedly insulin resistant and those that are not.

Finally, it is not logical that millions of people around the world are evolving to have resistance to a natural body hormone. The incidence of diabetes is increasing in every nation in the world. It does not make sense that some humans, but not all, in these countries are evolving in a very short time to be resistant to a natural body hormone that helps them utilize glucose as fuel for energy. Diabetes is not a contagious disease and no other hormones are being affected to the extent that we see among the increasing numbers of people developing diabetes.

I suggest you must also consider the illogical paradox of how modern medicine treats Type 2 diabetes for many patients: that is, with insulin injections. In no other disease, such as a bacterial infection, do doctors regularly prescribe an antibiotic that the patient is resistant to. For example, have you ever heard of a doctor prescribing even more penicillin to a patient with an infection who is resistant to penicillin? Yet, endocrinologists have for decades promoted and popularized the idea of using insulin for blood sugar control along with diet and exercise.

A final question to ponder: If insulin injections supposedly help people with Type 2 with strict control of their blood sugar level, why do so many of them incur the severe consequences of diabetes? Type 2 diabetics, even those on insulin, have a 50% chance of sustaining damage to kidney function, a 25% chance of complications related to vision, and an increased chance of sustaining complications related to the heart, blood vessels, limbs, and brain functions, compared to people without diabetes. In addition, there is 25% chance of developing complications associated with low blood sugar.

There is no question that sustained blood glucose elevation can lead to dangerous and even life-threatening condition, because excessive amounts of glucose can cause damage to various types of cells in the body, including nerve cells and cells in the blood vessels, heart, kidney, and eyes. However, the complications sustained by organs following damage to the cells lining the blood vessels come mainly from blockages caused by deposits of fat such as cholesterol and triglyceride. Most people are unaware that when you use insulin to lower your blood sugar level, the glucose removed from the blood is converted to these fat molecules, thus increasing your chances of blood vessel blockages, not lowering them.

This could explain why according to the National Institute of Diabetes and Digestive and Kidney Diseases, heart disease and stroke are the two leading causes of death among adults with diabetes. This is because narrow blood vessels make it harder for the heart to effectively pump oxygen-rich blood throughout the body. If a blood vessel leading to the brain gets blocked, it can lead to a stroke.

In fact, from 2017 to 2020, there were over one million deaths in the U.S. either directly due to Type 2 diabetes or from its being a contributing cause. Endocrinologists explain away these findings as the manifestations of the progressive nature of Type 2 diabetes, without clarifying why control of blood sugar with insulin injections did not prevent the progression of diabetes.

Why do you say that diabetes is a lifestyle condition?

In my view, Type 2 diabetes is clearly a lifestyle condition, not a hormonal disease. Consider a few examples that go a long way to proving that lifestyle is at the root of high blood sugar.

When Native Americans were moved to reservations in many states in the 1800s and 1900s, they often received complete physical examinations. The records of these show that from 1832–1939, Type 2 diabetes was extremely rare among Native Americans. However, after living on these reservations, Type 2 diabetes in Native Americans occurred in 16% of the population, compared to just 8% among Whites. It was clear that genetic changes did not explain this level of incidence. The most obvious cause was the lifestyle changes they experienced, particularly the profound dietary change Native Americans underwent in eating "westernized food," especially the grain-based complex carbohydrates that they were given on the reservations. Compare that to their ancestral way of living, when Native Americans did not cultivate grains but hunted, fished, and farmed crops other than grains like wheat.

There is also another study that supports the impact of grains in causing diabetes. In the 1970s, researcher Kerin O'Dea persuaded ten fully diabetic Aboriginal Australian people (five men and five women) with an average age of 54 to give up their urban diet and spend seven weeks living as hunter-gatherers in their traditional lands in northwestern Australia.

In the wild, they ate kangaroo meat, turtle, crocodile, fish, wild yams, and other foods, just like their forefathers had. While their urban diet had consisted of about 50% carbohydrates (from flour, rice, potatoes, sugared drinks, and alcohol), 40% fat from meat, and 10% protein, their diet in the wild averaged 61% protein, 24% fat, and only 16% carbohydrate.

The results of this seven-week experiment showed that every single participant had lowered their blood sugar to normal levels. While the researchers conducting this experiment believed that the reduced blood sugar levels were the result of the low-fat diet, I suggest that this experiment is more definitive proof that it is the reduction in carbohydrate consumption that leads to lower blood sugar—in as little as seven weeks. Dropping from 50% carbohydrate to just 16% carbohydrate in the diet is a much more significant change than that of fat intake in this experiment (from 40% to 24%). While many researchers in the 1970s were focused on the role of fat in causing heart disease, and rightfully so, we now know that the real source of that fat was the liver manufacturing it from excess glucose absorbed from the gut.

The results of a study of dietary changes in 18,090 adults by the Indian Council of Medical Research, published on August 27, 2022, give further evidence. The study had some of the adults eating a control diet consisting of 65–70% carbohydrates and little protein or fat. Meanwhile, the other adults had a diet consisting of 54–57% carbs, 16–20% protein, and 20–24% fat. This simple dietary change of reducing the daily carbohydrate intake by just 8–16%, mostly coming from eating less rice and wheat, resulted in significantly lowering blood sugar levels. This minimal dietary change is what can produce the results you are hoping for.

The current US guidelines for dietary changes for blood sugar control recommend reducing your intake of refined sugar, but this actually sidesteps the most significant source of blood sugar elevation in the modern day meal: complex carbohydrates from grain-based items. In fact. the dietary guidelines even encourage people to consume whole grains—the very food item that contains more glucose molecules than refined sugar, gram for gram.

This cookbook will familiarize you with the real types of food items you can prepare and enjoy without depending so much on grain-based complex carbohydrates, so you can avoid resorting to medications for your blood sugar control.

What is the connection between Type 2 diabetes, weight gain, and obesity?

In the United States, approximately 85% of people with Type 2 diabetes are overweight or obese. What is the connection? And which comes first—obesity or Type 2 diabetes?

According to the "insulin resistance" theory, it is suggested that the location of fat accumulation in the abdomen predisposes one to develop Type 2 diabetes. But to date, no one has demonstrated a difference in the type of fat stored in the abdominal fat cells vs. other fat cells in the body. Nor has anyone demonstrated that a difference in their metabolic functions among fat cells accounts for the development of Type 2 diabetes.

I have a different explanation for the association of weight gain and Type 2 diabetes. I suggest that weight gain occurs when adults consume an excess of calories that the body is then forced to store as fat. In the modern diet, the culprit in a high calorie diet is most often complex carbohydrates—grains and grain-flour foods—for some people, 50% or more of their daily caloric intake. When digested, complex carbohydrates release glucose that enters the bloodstream. After cells have absorbed however much glucose they need under the direction of insulin, the liver keeps a small amount in the form of glycogen, to be released back into the blood if the blood glucose level falls low, such as before lunch or dinner time. But the rest of the excess glucose is converted into fatty acids for long-term storage in our fat cells. If this fat is not burned off through exercise at some later time, it results in gradual weight gain—and eventually obesity.

Meanwhile, it also occurs in many overweight or obese individuals that their fat cell storage eventually fills up. When that happens, the fatty acids remain in circulation in the bloodstream and, as I have suggested, muscle cells begin using those fatty acids for their fuel rather than glucose. This is similar to a car with a hybrid engine using either gasoline or electricity to power the engine. I call this natural change the "fatty acid burn switch." The result: the burning of fatty acids leaves glucose in the bloodstream, leading to high blood sugar (hyperglycemia) and eventually a diagnosis of Type 2 diabetes.

This is the connection between obesity and Type 2 diabetes. Note, however, that even thin people can develop diabetes. This is because each person has a certain amount of fat storage capacity based on their body type. Thin people can equally fill up their smaller amount fat cells and, while they do not become obese, they may equally develop Type 2 diabetes when their fat storage capacity is filled, leaving glucose in the blood. The same mechanism can also explain gestational diabetes that affects 10% of pregnant women.

Does reducing body weight lead to lower blood sugar?

There is no question that reducing body weight leads to lower blood sugar levels. This is a recognized fact in the traditional treatment of Type 2 diabetes, although endocrinologists cannot explain why. While they claim that being overweight triggers insulin resistance, they are unable to explain the reverse, because they will not say that insulin resistance disappears if you lose weight.

Under my theory on the cause of Type 2 diabetes, the connection becomes clear. By losing weight, you empty your fat cells of fatty acids that are utilized for cellular energy.

Eventually, your muscle cells will begin functioning by burning glucose, lowering your blood sugar.

How much weight do you need to lose to begin lowering your blood sugar? I believe that the body has a natural "zone" of balance in which it functions at optimum levels to keep your blood sugar at the right level while providing you with enough energy for your daily functions. I call this zone your "authentic weight." If you are overweight or obese, getting back to your authentic weight and maintaining it requires you to moderate your food intake to the amount of calories that your body can use before the next meal.

How can you know this? In my view, each of us truly has a sense of our authentic weight because our brain tells us what it should be. Let me ask you right now: what is your authentic weight? If you focus on answering the question, it is likely that you can get a good sense of what you should weigh. Paying attention to your authentic weight is your brain's way of signaling that you are healthy, or that you are exceeding the weight that is right for you. When you are in tune with your authentic weight, you immediately know it if you gain a few extra pounds. You start to feel uncomfortable; you sense your gut is pulling on your muscles. You feel sluggish and tired.

In my view, you cannot rely on standardized tables of height and weight to know your authentic weight. Standardized weight tables are based on average weights of thousands of people and usually have a wide range of pounds in each weight category. How can you know whether you should be at the lower or the upper end of that range?

Nor can you count on your BMI (body mass index) to determine your weight. Your authentic body weight is a measure of the total mass of all components of your body, including bone, muscle, organs, blood, fat, and water. The role of each of these components of the body in contributing to one's weight differs in every individual in the world. Two people—one tall and small-boned with lots of muscle and another short and big-boned with regular muscle—could weigh the same. Only you can intuitively know your authentic weight based on what your brain assesses. Your authentic weight can also change as you exercise and age, because the contributions of each component of weight can change. If you begin working out, adding muscle, you might gain muscle weight but your brain knows you are still in your authentic range because it considers your extra muscle mass. If you are aging and losing muscle, but gain 10 pounds in body fat, your brain will sense that your authentic weight is now largely composed of fat, even though you may weigh the same.

To avoid Type 2 diabetes, your goal must be to take back control of your body and reclaim your authentic weight. If you are unable to rediscover your authentic weight, you can consider the body weight you had when you were in your mid-20s as a close approximation of it, provided your blood sugar and triglyceride levels were within normal range at that time. That is the age at which you probably reached your full height and your bones reached their maximum density. Any weight gain since that age will reflect in general the increase in pounds you have added due to storing fat and/or building muscle. (For most people, as they age, weight gain is due to storing fat!)

Why do people overeat?

Nearly all weight loss programs are based on the same premise: cut down your intake of food calories and/or increase your exercise in order to burn more calories. Effectively, they all use the same calories-in/calories-out approach.

This can be effective for some people for some amount of time, but it does not work for everyone. Even for those people who achieve their weight loss goal, it usually does not stick for the long term. They have cravings for foods that they really enjoyed in the past, or they travel and want to try new foods, or they attend parties and family get-togethers where it is almost impossible to resist eating, regardless of their will power. Gradually they fall back to the old way of eating and regain the weight they lost, and perhaps gain even more.

I suggest it helps to understand and reflect seriously on why you are tempted to eat more food than your body needs from meal to meal. This means that you have to pay attention to the reason you decide to eat any meal, however small it may be. Read the three reasons people overeat below and think about whether you are prone to any of these rather than eating only when your body sends you the hunger signal (which I discuss following these three reasons).

1. Eating for the pure enjoyment of it, even when you are not hungry. I suggest that non-hunger eating begins as a temporary and occasional event, done without recognizing its long-range significance. It then becomes a habit based on one's enjoyment of food, an experience that triggers the brain to generate dopamine, the pleasure hormone. Here's what happens.

In many adults, the habit of overeating starts as incidental to other events, such as family picnics or holiday dinners, or any other social occasion with others. It is not a deliberate act of overeating, but a random occurrence. The brain makes a connection between eating and enjoyment. The more these "extra" eating events occur in one's early life, the more that connection is reinforced. Whether you are hungry or not, if food is available and appealing, you learn to feel that it is okay to eat it without any consequences.

Little by little, you begin to rationalize overeating in these circumstances. The enjoyment of discovering new foods and the pleasure of eating them, as well as the association of food with positive memories, eventually overcomes your natural inclination to wait to eat until you truly feel hungry. In this way, you begin to establish a behavior of eating when simply stimulated by the sight, smell, or even just the thought of food rather than by your body's hunger signals. The connection between food and enjoyment is stored in your memory and expresses itself without any conscious or deliberate effort. Smelling food cooking, walking into a colorful supermarket, passing by a restaurant—all these trigger a pleasurable feeling caused by the release of the neurohormone *dopamine,* and you are prompted to want food. You look forward to enjoying a variety of good quality, tasty foods. Or you get a craving for one food in particular.

Once this rationale is established, even your awareness of potential adverse long-term consequences such as weight gain, high blood sugar, high blood cholesterol, or high blood pressure may not be a sufficient deterrent to prevent you from overeating. The behavior continues, even when the consequences are damaging.

2. Eating when hungry at first, then overeating until your stomach feels full. You may start eating in response to the sensation of hunger but rather than stopping when your hunger is satisfied, you don't stop eating until your stomach feels full and almost uncomfortable. You may have started this way accidentally by overeating at family events, parties, business meetings, or trips to new places where food is inexpensive or you are allowed to eat all you can for the same price. Think about it: most people don't drink until their stomach is full; they stop when their thirst is quenched. But the more times you eat until you feel full, rather than satiated, the more you begin to expect that full feeling. Overeating ensues and it becomes harder to achieve and maintain your authentic weight.

3. Eating to relieve stress and anxiety. Stress is any stimulus that you consider harmful to your safety, security, and wellbeing. People often experience stress as the result of two powerful feelings: fear and pain. This in turn induces the stress response that results in the release of hormones such as adrenaline and cortisol. Eating food can lower the amount of adrenaline released, and thus a person who is stressed may turn to food to mitigate the unpleasant effects of stress in the body.

People who tend to overeat often do so for two or three of these reasons rather than just one. The commonality between these is that they all demonstrate that when we overeat, we override the brain's hunger and satisfaction signals.

What are the body's hunger and satiation mechanisms?

To understand hunger, you don't need to look any farther than the mechanism by which babies regulate their consumption of milk, or toddlers regulate their consumption of food. If you think about it, both infants and toddlers decide on their own when to eat, what to eat, and how much to eat to thrive physically, mentally, and emotionally. When you were an infant and then a toddler, this is what you did. So today, to lose weight, you need to alter your eating habits so you can eat as you did decades ago. I call it "eating like a toddler."

Infants and toddlers only eat in response to the "hunger signal." And they stop eating in response to the "satiation signal." They do not keep eating even if there is food left on the plate. Let me define these two signals.

Hunger signal. Have you ever wondered about the fact that you can never predict precisely when you are going to feel hungry? You probably know, logically and from experience, that you tend to eat every few hours, but what causes the brain to generate the actual sensation of hunger? I suggest that hunger is the feeling that the brain produces to indicate when your body needs nutrients. However, with the body needing over 100 different nutrients for healthy functioning, what makes the brain decide when to create the sensation of hunger?

In my view, it is likely that the brain is responding to cells throughout the body calling for a variety of nutrients, not just a single nutrient. When the total need of nutrients reaches some threshold level, the brain generates that very recognizable sensation of hunger you feel. To lose weight, see if you can avoid eating until you truly feel the pangs of hunger.

Satiation signal. As I mentioned, we usually do not drink liquids until our stomach is full. We stop drinking when our thirst is quenched, according to a signal the brain send us. Similarly, the brain actually sends us a signal that we have eaten enough. If you pay attention to chewing your food, you will notice that the taste of the food you are eating becomes less and less enjoyable. This is the brain telling you that it has received enough nutrients for the present moment.

The problem is, most of us get used to eating until our stomach is full. Even if we are not enjoying the food as much as those first bites, we keep eating until the stomach sends a signal to the brain, saying the equivalent of "Enough, I can't digest any more, please stop." This is effectively a backup signal that the brain sends to stop eating.

Why do so many people disregard the loss of enjoyment signal and keep eating until the full stomach signal alerts them? In my view, it has to do with the habit of overeating we develop—for any or all of the three reasons cited above—in our youth, when there appear to be no consequences. We are not usually gaining much weight at that age, nor incurring high blood sugar, so we start believing that overeating is okay once in a while. Then it becomes a regular eating pattern.

To lose weight, you must therefore become conscious of when you are truly hungry and when your brain is signaling you to stop eating. Think, as I said, that you need to start "eating like a toddler."

I want to make the transition from grains, but what can I eat?

The ancestors of modern humans appeared on earth about 50,000 years ago. Cultivation of plants started only after 40,000 years of human existence. The domestication of rice and grains like wheat and rye dates to only about 13,000–10,000 BCE. This means that humans survived without consuming significant amounts of grain and grain products for the majority of human life on earth.

Humans were always equipped to break down complex carbohydrates. But it's likely that early humans obtained complex carbohydrates and carbohydrate-associated nutrients from vegetables that required chewing, such as yam, cassava, potato, and taro. It was not until several millennia ago that carbohydrates from grains became a staple of the human diet. In the Middle Ages, many cultures survived on porridge, rice, or potatoes, depending on which of these crops grew in their region. In the late 19th century, industrialized roller mills were invented, making it easier to refine grains into flour and other products made with starches and flours. Largely because of this, grains became the major source of carbohydrates in human diets.

Over the last century, as never before, modern agricultural practices have increased grain cultivation and the production of grain products, fueling a tremendous increase in the role of grains in our diets. Today, grains have become very easy to transport, are fast to cook, easy to chew, and are relatively easily digested and absorbed (except by people with celiac disease or grain allergies). Milling grains to create flour makes them easy to store without refrigeration. The variety of edible products that can be made with the carbohydrate from grains is never-ending, and these food items tempt people throughout the world. Carbohydrate intake from grains now accounts for over 50% of the calories in the typical adult diet in the US.

If you are going to eat grains, I suggest that you emphasize alternatives to wheat, rice, and corn. The table here shows you how much carbohydrate, fiber, fat, and protein (in grams) is contained in a variety of grains per 100 grams.

Grain	Carbohydrate	Fiber content	Fat content	Protein
White rice	91	1	1	7
Wheat	82	1.2	1.5	12.6
Corn	82	3	1	3
Oats	66	11.6	6.9	16.9
Quinoa	64	7	1.9	14.1
Millet	54	22.6	1.0	7.4

As you can see, if you begin substituting oats, quinoa, and millet in your diet for wheat, rice, and corn, you will obtain the benefits of less carbohydrate, more fiber, more fat, and more protein.

Once you become comfortable with the above, you can attempt further reduction of complex carbohydrate by substituting the following whenever possible.

- **Almond flour.** With a consistency like corn meal, almond flour can be used in pastry, confectionary, and other baking items. Per 100 grams, almond flour contains 21.6 g carbohydrates, 12.5 g dietary fiber, 49.9 g fat, and 21.2 g protein.

- **Chickpea flour.** Also known as besan, this is a pulse flour made from a variety of ground chickpea called Bengal gram or kaalachana. Per 100 grams, it contains 57 g carbohydrates, 10 g dietary fiber, 6 g fat and 22 g protein.

- **Cauliflower flour.** This is an alternative to rice flour. Per 100 grams, it contains 5 g carbohydrates, 2 g dietary fiber, 0.3 g fat and 1.9 g protein.

What other practical suggestions do you have for things I can do to lose weight?

I recommend the following simple changes to your eating habits:

1. As much as possible, during each meal, eat food items that require chewing. Studies suggest that increasing the number of chews per bite increases relevant intestinal signals and may decrease self-reported hunger and food intake. In other words, continued chewing sends more signals from the mouth to the food intake control centers in the brain, facilitating more enjoyment related to that food, and later leading to moderation of the intensity of hunger, thus creating the feeling of satisfaction that allows you to terminate the act of eating and reduce total food energy intake.

2. Sipping warm water every few minutes during a meal cleans the taste buds, creating more contact points for nutrient registration and signal generation to the brain.

3. Concentrate on vegetable preparations that need chewing, rather than blended and pureed foods which do not allow for chewing.

4. To increase chewing, add nuts to certain dishes, or serve on the side.

5. Severely limit the consumption of refined grains and food items made with refined grain-flour that require practically no chewing. From a nutritional point of

view, foods made with refined grains and refined grain-flour are empty-calorie foods. If you plan to eat grains or grain-flour-based foods, use whole grain products instead. To reduce the consumption of glucose-releasing foods, limit the intake of grain-based food items such as bread, rolls, pasta, cookies, cakes, etc. to not more than 200 of the 570 calories of a single meal.

6. Prepare food items you plan to eat at home, rather than buying pre-made or pre-packaged. This will give you a head start to limit your intake of total daily food energy and grain-based food items. An additional benefit is limiting your intake of salt.

What causes weight regain after weight loss?

In general, weight reduction programs that include individual or group counseling to modify how much you eat result in only a 5–10% weight loss. Unfortunately, the statistics show that, after six to twelve months following the completion of such a program, most people start regaining the weight.

Experts suggest many possible reasons for this finding, though they seldom provide any evidence. For example, one theory states that weight loss reduces the rate at which your body burns calories. This then, the theory says, makes it difficult to lose more weight over a period of months. That seems illogical, however, as it implies that losing weight has a cap on how much can be lost.

Other theories suggest that a rate of weight loss larger than one-half to two pounds per week results in the failure of long-term maintenance of reduced weight. For example, most people who lose weight rapidly or a large amount of weight have regained it two to three years later. But why? The theorists do not explain it.

Let me suggest a few possible logical reasons for regaining lost weight. First, let's consider motivation. It is normal to be enthusiastic about any new endeavor, and that enthusiasm makes it easy to commit to a goal. Losing weight as part of an organized program helps motivate you to accomplish your objective. However, over time you may find you gradually begin to miss the way you were eating before, or the type and quantity of food you used to eat, so you slide back into your former way of eating, regaining the lost weight. This is de-motivating and a real challenge to your sense of commitment.

If you lost weight with the help of medications that modified your natural control mechanisms, terminating the medications could cause a reset of the brain's control mechanisms regarding how hungry you feel and how much you need to eat. This can then result in regaining the lost weight.

The best way to avoid regaining weight is, as explained above, to remain conscious of why you are eating. Are you truly hungry? Or are you eating out of a need to enjoy food, or out of stress or other emotions, or eating until your stomach feels full rather than being truly satiated?

I also suggest you build the following habits into your daily routine. Check your weight every day around the same time and adjust your food intake for the next 24 hours based on noticing any weight gain. Be aware that you sometimes will have unexpected weight swings due to an excess intake of salt. This causes your body to retain water in order to keep the salt concentration optimal for proper cellular functioning. For this reason, many programs will advise you to weigh yourself no more often than every few days, or only once a week or month. However, it is important to check your weight every day in order to see potential issues as soon as possible.

Take pride in yourself when you have a day that shows no weight gain. Notice what you ate the day before that helped you avoid putting on a pound or two. If you put on weight, try eating a large salad for lunch or dinner in place of your usual big meal to lose that extra pound you gained the day before.

Of course, I do agree that it's okay to allow yourself to have an occasional large meal now and again if you have an event or holiday gathering. But if you know you are going to overeat at an event, preplan and adjust your food intake during the few days before it. And always be aware of your intake of grains.

What is the connection between a sedentary lifestyle and diabetes?

Experts suggest that sedentary lifestyle and dietary habits are the major factors for the rising incidence of Type 2 diabetes.

A study carried out for a period of six years among more than a thousand nondiabetic individuals from the high-risk population of Pima Indians found that the diabetes incidence rate remained higher in less active men and women from all BMI groups.

Experts suggest that reduced insulin sensitivity in physically less active people leads to the development of diabetes. However, there is no clear explanation of the mechanism by which physical inactivity contributes to the development of Type 2 diabetes.

On the other hand, a CDC report showed that in 2018 there were 28 million people between ages 18–44 diagnosed with prediabetes compared to 24 million people above age 65 in the United States. If physical inactivity was a significant contributor to the development of diabetes, this finding should have been reversed, showing a higher incidence of Type 2 diabetes among the older people. In addition, if it were true that less active people develop insulin insensitivity and diabetes, nearly all elderly people living in retirement facilities should be diabetic or at least prediabetic. But there is no evidence to show this is the case.

In my view, the link between a sedentary lifestyle and diabetes is related to the theory I have proposed as the cause of Type 2 diabetes. As this book has suggested, a diet high in grains creates voluminous amounts of glucose in the bloodstream. Any glucose that the body does not utilize immediately (within hours of digesting food) is converted to fatty acids that need to be stored in the fat cells for later use. When the fat cells become full, however, further excess fatty acids remain the bloodstream, to become the primary fuel for muscle cells.

However, if you are sedentary, your muscle cells are not utilizing those fatty acids, but neither are they utilizing any glucose created from the foods you digest. The result is the same: excess glucose in the bloodstream, hence one initially develops high blood sugar (pre-diabetes) and eventually Type 2 diabetes. In both cases, the real cause is a diet high in grains and grain-flour products. As to why not all elderly people develop diabetes given that they are largely sedentary, the answer is simply that they tend to eat less. It is universally known that the older one gets, the more one's appetite decreases as the body seems to naturally accommodate to less activity.

Why do we need to eat a variety of foods?

Human beings moved from their place of birth to different areas in different continents either to escape inclement living conditions or to reach more favorable living conditions. By surviving in various parts of the earth, humans revealed that there is an abundant availability of nutrients on a timely basis in sufficient quantities for healthy living. In short, nature has made it possible for humans to survive in almost every part of the globe.

Almost all natural foods from which humans can acquire nutrients come in "containers" made of organic molecules such as cellulose. Think fruits, vegetables, and nuts. Nature appears to have made these forms of packaging not only to preserve nutrients for the long term, but also to protect food from predators. The packaging in different parts of the globe is different in size, shape, color, aroma, texture, and flavor.

The body needs many nutrients for normal functioning. Science has identified 118 nutrients that are used at some time for human health. No one knows with certainty how much of each of these the body needs or how we derive them from the foods we eat. That is why I always suggest eating a wide variety of foods to ensure you have the opportunity to ingest as many of these nutrients as possible. It is also why I do not believe in fixed diets or third-party programs that supply you with your meals. Only your brain can tell you what you need to eat.

Do artificial sweeteners help control blood sugar?

People with Type 2 diabetes often avoid natural sugar and use artificial sweeteners to lose weight and reduce their blood sugar level. This could be counterproductive. Let me explain.

When nutrients such as natural sugar are detected by the receptors in the oral cavity, two alerts are sent: one to the food intake control centers in the brain and the second to the intestine. The brain rewards you by generating the sensation of enjoyment, based on the need for that nutrient in your body at that time. When food reaches the intestine, signals go to the brain, which, in turn, reduces the intensity of enjoyment related to the incoming nutrients to prevent overeating.

Artificial sweeteners, on the other hand, can trigger the sensation of sweet taste. However, they don't appear to be effective in moderating food intake. In fact, evidence shows that long-term use of aspartame, sucralose, stevia, and saccharin leads to weight gain and higher blood sugar levels. This suggests that while the enjoyment of a natural nutrient such as sugar is based on satisfaction of obtaining a useful nutrient, the sensation felt with artificial sweetener appears to be based on a conditioned reflex reacting to sweetness from previous experiences. This conditioned response could also explain why some people addicted to artificial sweeteners can't enjoy natural sweetness of fruits without adding artificial sweeteners to them.

Erythritol, a popular artificial sweetener used in many sugar-free food products, has been linked to increased risk of heart attacks and strokes, according to an article in the February 2023 issue of *Nature Medicine*.[8] Erythritol is found in very small amounts in fruits and vegetables and is excreted from the body in urine, unchanged. People assume that erythritol is safe because it occurs in nature. However, the quantity added to a prepared food can be 1,000 times greater than that seen in natural foods.

The fact is, the natural sugar consumed on average in everyday drinks and foods is not a significant contributor to blood sugar, unless you drink a large amount of soft drinks sweetened with sugar. The main cause of blood sugar elevation in Type 2 diabetes is glucose released after the digestion of complex carbohydrates in grains such as wheat, rice, and corn. Therefore, if you can cut the amount of grain-based foods to one-half of what you are consuming on a daily basis, you can lower your blood sugar and continue to enjoy natural table sugar in your tea, coffee, and your food preparations.

Is natural sugar bad for diabetics?

Many people are confused about whether natural sugar, i.e., sucrose, is the same as glucose in your bloodstream. Sucrose is found in fruit, berries, sugar cane, sugar beets, and other

---

8. The artificial sweetener erythritol and cardiovascular event risk. M. Witkowski, I. Nemet, H. Alamri, et al: Nature Medicine: Feb 2023

crops that can be boiled down into forms of sugar. The confusion is understandable because, when discussing diabetes, we always refer to the problem of having high blood "sugar." The same word "sugar" appears to be referring to the same item, so there is a tendency to think that eating any natural sugar increases your blood sugar.

For example, many people make pastries with reduced amounts of sugar (sucrose), believing that they can now consume more of the pastries, without realizing that these are likely contributing more sugar (glucose) from the flour used than the natural sugar in their coffee.

Digesting natural sugar (sucrose) is not the same as filling your bloodstream with glucose. Sucrose contains equal parts of glucose and fructose. Both are absorbed as they're released in the intestine. But while the glucose adds to your blood sugar level almost immediately, fructose is absorbed only half as fast as glucose and has to be further processed into glucose before it can elevate your blood sugar level. This means eating a piece of fruit for breakfast or dessert doesn't cause the same level of blood sugar peak compared to an equal amount of carbohydrate in a grain-based product such as toast, muffins, cake, or pie, so it is effectively healthier for you.

The same is true for milk sugar (lactose), which is made of one molecule of galactose and one molecule of glucose. Galactose must be further processed by the liver before it can elevate your blood sugar. The medical profession has done a poor job of educating people that natural sugar has not been shown to increase the incidence of complications in Type 2 diabetes. In fact, the medical profession may have unwittingly contributed to creating a prevailing culture in which people fear the natural sugars of whole fruit.

Should I eat according to the 2023 Food Pyramid?

The first Food Pyramid was created in the 1970s in Sweden by a special committee to suggest nutritionally balanced meals at a reasonable cost. In 1992 the United States Department of Agriculture (USDA) introduced a Food Pyramid to recommend servings of each food group, which previous guides did not do.

The 2023 Food Pyramid modified the recommendations in an attempt to improve the health of Americans who continued to experience increasing incidence of cardiovascular diseases and Type 2 diabetes. For example, meats are to be consumed monthly or in small amounts compared to the previous recommendation of 2 to 3 servings per day. Eggs, poultry, and dairy are to be taken daily to weekly, compared to prior recommendation of 2 to 3 servings a day. Fish and seafood are to be eaten a few times per week compared to 2 to 3 times per day. Olive oil can be consumed in variable amounts daily compared to sparingly. Fruits and vegetables can be consumed daily compared 3 to 5 servings per day. Whole grains, bread, legumes and nuts can be taken daily compared to 6 to 11 servings per day of bread, cereal, rice, and pasta.

In essence, the new Food Pyramid is primarily based on the Mediterranean diet. Overall, that diet is mostly plant-based and focuses on healthy fats that include virgin olive oil, avocados, nuts, salmon, and sardines. Red meat consumption is limited to a few times a month.

As you can see, the emphasis of both pyramids, the original and the new USDA version, is on minimizing the intake of dietary fat, especially saturated fat such as cholesterol, that literally creates the plaque that blocks blood passages and leads to heart attacks and strokes.

However, in my opinion the new pyramid will not help achieve the objective of reducing the incidence of cardiovascular events or Type 2 diabetes. This is because it fails to address the root cause of excess food consumption. In addition, the investigators failed to take into consideration that vegetarians who do not consume animal products also get the same cardiovascular diseases. Even more importantly, although the calculation of average intake of food groups can be useful for comparison of study results, it cannot be directly applicable to all individuals because each person's nutrient needs are different.

This major deficiency is what I am trying to offset in this book in order to reverse and prevent Type 2 diabetes through my recommendations. Exercise, weight control, and reducing the consumption of grains and grain-flour products are the essential keys to avoiding Type 2 diabetes and its myriad complications.

Can meal timing help with weight control?

An estimated 33% of the global adult population is classified as overweight. Some researchers looking to lower this number think that "meal timing" can be a viable solution to helping people lose weight.

In some short-duration studies (5–6 weeks only), it has been shown that participants with a high degree of compliance were able to control their weight by consuming more calories in the morning than during the later part of the day. The research suggests that our bodies are primed to metabolize food after the overnight fasting period, and therefore we should eat the majority of our calories during the morning or afternoon. The recommendations also emphasize not to skip breakfast as it could lead to more intense hunger and binge eating later in the day.

Another suggestion is to eat a small dinner early in the evening or at least two to three hours before going to bed. In general, researchers recommend eating this way at least five times a week if it is not possible to do it daily. Researchers claim that these recommendations are based on the natural biological clock in the body that activates physiological mechanisms, including those related to hunger and food intake.

However, I suggest that one does not need to gorge oneself at breakfast. It is understandable that the body activates the hunger mechanism after sleeping due to a need to replenish nutrients, but it is also obvious that the body is not expecting a sudden influx of nutrients, otherwise one would feel the greatest intensity of hunger in the morning, which for most people, is not so. The fact that the hunger sensation can be felt at any time of the day means that the body can handle eating for nutrition whenever it is ready for it, regardless of time of the day.

An extreme example of meal timing is intermittent fasting to reduce food calorie intake by eating only alternate days, not eating certain days of the week, or restricting eating to specified times of the day. Although considered harmless, the US National Institute on Aging states that there is insufficient evidence to recommend intermittent fasting for general use. A study published in the *Journal of the American Heart Association* in 2023 concluded that the use of time-determined eating was not helpful as a strategy for long-term weight loss in a general medical population.[9]

Can I have a surgical procedure to lose weight?

In extreme cases, medical practitioners may suggest bariatric surgery, pointing out that most people maintain reduced weight after the surgery. But most such surgical procedures achieve long-term weight loss through one of three mechanisms: decreasing nutrient absorption, restricting food intake, or affecting the body's cell signaling pathways. Often, the procedures affect several of these mechanisms. Let me explain them.

Some procedures reduce the ability of the intestines to absorb nutrients. Though this may help a person lose weight, it can also result in deficiencies of iron, vitamin B12, fat soluble vitamins, thiamine, and folate. Inappropriate insulin secretion is another complication of this type of surgery. Yet another complication is deep vein thrombosis with a potential for pulmonary embolism. In addition, rapid weight loss after obesity surgery can contribute to the development of gallstones. Increased incidence of alcohol and mental health related issues have been reported after obesity surgery.

Other procedures restrict your food intake by making the stomach smaller. The gastric bypass, one of the common bariatric surgeries, reduces the size of the stomach by well over 90% to about 15 milliliter (mL) in size compared to a normal stomach that can stretch, sometimes to over 1000 mL. What you may not realize is that this procedure helps you lose weight simply because you cannot eat as much as before. So before agreeing to this type of surgery, I suggest you find out how much food someone who had this type of surgery can consume. Then consume a similar amount of food for a while. See if you can achieve similar weight loss and weight maintenance without having to suffer the surgery or its consequences.

---

9. ahajournals.org/doi/10.1161/JAHA.122.026484

Another procedure is thought to affect weight loss by altering the physiology of weight regulation and eating behavior. For example, after surgery, patients are asked to have 5–6 small meals daily, and *not* graze between meals. Meals after surgery are restricted to only ¼–½ cup, slowly increasing to 1 cup over the span of one year.

A warning, as well: after bariatric surgery, people may tend to feel good about themselves for the weight loss, but a significant minority experience psychological complications, including but not limited to grieving the loss of food, regrets about having had surgery, relationship changes, and fear of weight regain. One study that followed up for nearly 40 years on almost 22,000 surgical patients representing the major types of bariatric surgeries showed a reduction in mortality rates, including cardiovascular-, cancer-, and diabetes-related death rates compared to matching controls. However, patients in that study between ages 18–34 had increased mortality following bariatric surgery in relation to suicide, accidents, and cirrhosis of the liver. The authors of the study recommended more research in these areas.

Why can't I take insulin or other drugs to control my blood sugar?

You can use insulin to control your blood sugar and you might believe that it will help you escape the usual complications of Type 2 diabetes in the long term. But what may be surprising for most Type 2 diabetic patients is the fact that even if you keep your blood sugar below 7 as indicated by your A1C, you are still likely to develop kidney function failure and increased chances of developing heart, brain, vision, and leg problems, compared to controlling your blood sugar with dietary changes.

Other drugs currently used to control blood sugar work by prolonging the action of the intestinal signaling mechanisms that control your desire for food intake. For example, the intestine releases a hormone in response to glucose molecules in food as soon as you start eating. This hormone then stimulates the pancreas to release insulin to help digest glucose. The hormone also promotes brain action to suppress the sensation of hunger, which is usually degraded within minutes.

Pharmaceutical researchers have therefore found a way to prolong the action of this intestinal hormone so that it continues to stimulate insulin release and thus a longer suppression of hunger. However, these drugs often cause nausea, vomiting, diarrhea, and constipation in a significant number of people. It is understandable that people with upset stomach will take less food and lose weight.

Meanwhile, the use of weight loss drugs to control appetite also carries many side effects, one of which is interference with the absorption of necessary nutrients in a timely fashion, which can lead to food cravings.

Will changing my diet increase my lifespan?

It is well recognized that Type 2 diabetes is associated with an overall shorter lifespan. For example, just by reducing A1C (hemoglobin blood sugar) from 9.9% to 7.7%, it has been shown that you might gain 3.4 years in life expectancy.

What is even more worrisome is that as the age of people diagnosed with Type 2 diabetes goes down (now even occurring in teens and pre-teens), we can expect a further gradual decrease in lifespan. Unfortunately, diabetologists have no specific strategies to address the increasing incidence of diabetes occurring at younger and younger ages. This is a true tragedy.

As discussed earlier, the metabolic activities inside each cell in the body produce agents known as "Reactive Oxygen Species" (ROS). These agents can cause damage to proteins and/or the genes inside the cell. This is what causes an age-related limit on lifespan due to cellular damage.

There are four possible outcomes when cells sustain gene damage:

1. **Repair and maintenance.** Cells can actually repair damaged genes in their structure and functionality. The greater one's body is able to repair gene damage, the longer one's life span. It has been shown that centenarians 100–107 years old have greater levels of gene repair mechanisms compared to 69–75-year-old individuals in the general population.

2. **Defective functionality.** Without gene repair, the accumulation of damage to genes as humans age not only limits the functional capability of cells, which causes a reduced lifespan, but it also leads to a gradual reduction in the quality of life. This occurs because gene damage can limit muscle strength and stamina. One highly visible example of the result of such injury is hair loss as one ages due to gene damage sustained by stem cells in charge of hair renewal.

3. **Uncontrolled Activity:** The accumulation of gene damage can also result in uncontrolled cell multiplication, which initiates the formation of a cancer tumor. However, this usually occurs over an extended amount of time, literally decades. The average age of an adult cancer patient is over sixty years. (Note that gene damage resulting in cancer can also be due to factors other than ROS. For example, radiation, exposure to cancer-causing chemicals in cigarettes and in the environment, infections, and chronic inflammation can all lead to either damage to existing genes or mistakes during gene construction.)

4. **Cellular senescence.** When cells have accomplished their assigned tasks, they enter into a state of inactivity called cellular senescence (old age), after which cells

in the immune system clear them away. However, when the rate of generation of senescent cells exceeds the capability of the immune system to remove them, perhaps due to an age-related decline in immune function, senescent cells can persist. Although they may not be able to perform useful functions, they may remain metabolically active, producing molecules that promote inflammation. For example, scientists link an accumulation of senescent cells in lungs that were exposed to cigarette smoke as contributing to airway inflammation. Exercise has been shown to improve the efficiency of the immune system to remove senescent cells and improve muscle strength in older adults.

In summary, most age-related disabilities stem from the imbalance between cellular damage due to normal metabolic activities and the ability of the immune system to recognize and repair it. One solution is to reduce cellular metabolic activities, which will limit the production of ROS. The best example of how effective this can be is the lifespan of Greenland sharks, which—barring injury, poison, disease, lack of available resources, changes to environment, or capture—can live between 250 and 500 years. These sharks have the lowest swim speed and tail-beat frequency relative to their size across all fish species, which most likely correlates with their very slow metabolism and extreme longevity.

However, humans, because of our greater brain capabilities and continuous inputs from our senses, are compelled to engage in activities that create a large amount of ROS.

Nevertheless, there are some mitigating actions that you can take to lower the production of ROS. One significant step is to reduce stress, which helps reduce the production of ROS. With training and practice, you can learn to deal with a stressful event with minimal release of stress hormones. In addition, exercise can help you expend some of the stress hormones released, reducing their impact on metabolic activities that could lead to more ROS generation. Read about stress in the answer to the following question.

What is the role of stress in diabetes?

The word stress generally refers to a force or influence; as applied to the lives of humans, stress refers to any stimulus that alters the meaning or intensity of one's feelings, actions, or communications. Signals that you interpret as harmful to your safety, security, or wellbeing are the ones that cause a stress response. The stimuli that cause stress are essentially the same for most people—perceived threats, illness, injury, overwork, unsolved work issues, family problems, relationship issues, or inconveniences. The intensity and duration of the stimuli needed to elicit the stress response varies for each person. One individual may be able to handle many difficult life events that another would find highly stressful. The difference appears to be due to the conditioning and training one receives from parents to cope with stress starting in early childhood and continuing to adulthood which determines a person's sensitivity to stressful stimuli as an adult.

In general, people experience stress as two powerful feelings: fear or pain. Fear can be imagined or real and based on known or unforeseen factors. Fear, by definition, is more emotional than rational. During the fear response, neurons located in the primitive core part of the brain (the limbic system) are activated before the stimulus can be analyzed on the intellectual level (in the prefrontal cortex) to determine if it is real and deserves a thoughtful reaction. This fear forces you to determine what to do based on an incomplete analysis of partial information. Pain can be physical or emotional. It can be based on a current event or a past experience.

The time of onset, degree, and duration of the stress response varies with each individual, as determined by the hormones released in the body during the stress response. For instance, let's look at anger, a feeling of displeasure aroused by a real or imagined stress. If your body releases adrenaline at the slightest provocation, you're a person who will get angry quickly and easily. If the amount of adrenaline released is large or if your sensitivity to it is high, the intensity of your anger will also be high. If you remain in the stressful environment or dwell on the stress in your mind, your body can continue releasing the hormone for a long period, setting the stage for prolonged anger. If you routinely expect a person or event to create displeasure for you, it may cause you to be angry each time you encounter that person or event.

The role of stress in diabetes is related to two consequences. First, when you are under stress you may react by eating, since the dopamine hormone released by the pleasures of eating can counterbalance the stress hormones and lessen the sensation of stress.

Secondly, just receiving a diagnosis of Type 2 diabetes can trigger a continuous sense of stress in many people. In my opinion, the quality of life deteriorates from the moment Type 2 diabetes is diagnosed. The patient is confused about the reason for getting diabetes. Doctors will usually ask about one's family history of diabetes, and the patient is more likely than not to conclude that it is hereditary because someone in the family has it now or had it. The patient will be asked to lose weight and given instructions not to skip meals while on diabetic medications lest she may suffer symptoms of low blood sugar.

This life change is often stressful for a person who has never experienced symptoms of low blood sugar and therefore is unfamiliar with what they are supposed to feel. A low-level sense of trepidation and fear may become common in the person's life. They may not know what to do when they feel a sharp hunger sensation as a consequence of taking the diabetic medication. Meanwhile, to prevent the consequences of low blood sugar, the doctor may have advised the patient to carry food at all times, especially when access to sugar-containing food is not assured, such as when traveling. Family members and friends may worry about not being able to serve what the person is allowed to eat, or worse, not knowing how to deal with a low blood sugar situation if it occurs. Gradually, the person who has been diagnosed with Type 2 diabetes may decline to go out very much for fear of inconveniencing their friends and family. This could lead to emotional distress and its related stress responses, thus creating further doubts about being able to control one's diabetes.

How does exercise improve the quality of life?

Remaining physically active as we grow old is the best way to prevent or keep in check lifestyle-related illnesses like diabetes in order to maintain the quality of life and increase one's lifespan. A key indicator of the state of one's physical health is the efficiency of the metabolic activities inside each cell. Aging naturally affects that efficiency, by reducing the power generation of mitochondria, which leads to more ROS production. This, in turn, not only increases the chance of lifestyle-associated diseases but also accelerates the aging process. This is precisely why exercise is critical to your quality of life. It has been shown that lifelong exercise training improves mitochondrial efficiency, lowers ROS production, and contributes to healthy aging.

There are many additional health benefits from regular exercise that affect the quality of life. For example, chances are you have never thought about how blood returns to the heart from different parts of the body, even against gravity, for example, from the legs, compared to the heart sending it there by the force of the heartbeat. You may not realize that the return of blood is aided by contractions of muscles that act as pumps to push the blood through the veins. To prevent blood from dropping back under the pull of gravity, veins have valves spaced at different intervals. It is when these valves fail that you see the bulging that creates varicose veins. In addition, if you remain immobile for extended periods of time, such as during air travel or if you are bedridden, blood can stay stagnant, leading to the formation of blood clots that can be dangerous.

To help you with your decision to exercise regularly, let me give you a few suggestions:

1. **Be clear about why you want to exercise and what your exact objective is.** For example, you might want to feel good about yourself being able to continue and enjoy certain physical activities as long as you can. Or you may want to improve your stamina or build muscle in order to keep up with your grandchildren. Perhaps you simply want to be able to carry out your everyday tasks, such as getting in and out of a car, more easily.

2. **Be adaptive.** Sometimes you may find it hard to exercise because of travel, illness, or a pressing need for your time; rather than letting this situation discourage you, be adaptive and look forward to the next chance.

3. **Connect exercise with something you routinely do.** For example, consider exercising every morning after your personal hygiene needs are met or before you settle down in the evening in front of the television.

4. **Appreciate your ability to continue physical exercise.** Patting yourself on the back is both a good literal and motivational exercise.

To make physical exercise a part of your daily routine, start slowly, especially if you have been relatively sedentary for a long time. Create a mindset of curiosity to understand what the exercise you plan to do is about and how it can help you. As you gradually master each exercise routine, you will find it increasingly comfortable to do. You will notice positive impacts in all aspects of your life. With commitment and perseverance, you will begin looking forward to exercising and even miss it when you can't do it due to travel or other pressing needs.

ABOUT THE AUTHORS

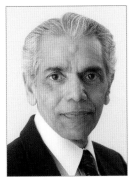

John M. Poothullil, MD, FRCP

Dr. Poothullil practiced medicine as a pediatrician and allergist for more than 30 years, with 27 of those years in the state of Texas. He received his medical degree from the University of Kerala, India in 1968, after which he completed two years of medical residency in Washington, D.C., and Phoenix, Arizona and two years of fellowship, one in Milwaukee, Wisconsin and the other in Ontario, Canada. He began his practice in 1974 and retired in 2008. He holds certifications from the American Board of Pediatrics, The American Board of Allergy & Immunology, and the Canadian Board of Pediatrics.

During his medical practice, John became interested in understanding the causes of and interconnections between hunger, satiation, and weight gain. His interest turned into a passion and a multi-decade personal study and research project that led him to read many medical journal articles, medical textbooks, and other scholarly works in biology, biochemistry, physiology, endocrinology, and cellular metabolic functions. This eventually guided Dr. Poothullil to investigate the theory of insulin resistance as it relates to diabetes. Recognizing that this theory was illogical, he spent several years rethinking the biology behind high blood sugar and developed the fatty acid burn theory as the real cause of diabetes.

He then continued researching the linkage between diabetes and cancer and developed additional insights into the causes of childhood and adult cancer and possible treatments involving low-carbohydrate diets to initiate starving of cancer cells by removing their main source of energy—glucose from grains.

Dr. Poothullil has written articles on hunger and satiation, weight loss, diabetes, and the senses of taste and smell. His articles have been published in medical journals such as *Physiology and Behavior*, *Neuroscience and Biobehavioral Reviews*, *Journal of Women's Health*, *Journal of Applied Research*, *Nutrition*, and *Nutritional Neuroscience*. His articles on diabetes have been published in *Alternative Medicine*, *Whole Person*, *India Abroad*, and several other magazines.

Dr. Poothullil is an active speaker on diabetes and cancer. He has appeared on four television shows, interviewed on over 60 national and local radio programs, and given more than 40 talks to groups in bookstores and private groups and associations. An interview with him appeared in the *Washington Post*. He has published nearly 130 blogs on his website DrJohnOnHealth.com.

In addition to his two books on diabetes and his book on medical disinformation (see Other Books By Dr. John Poothullil page), he has written two books on cancer:

• *Surviving Cancer: A New Perspective on Why Cancer Happens & Your Key Strategies for a Healthy Life* (New Insights Press, 2017)

• *When Your Child Has Cancer: Insights and Information to Empower Parents* (New Insights Press, 2020)

Chef Colleen Cackowski

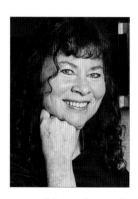

In 1996, Colleen walked into a health food store while a demonstration was going on with a chef who had worked at Gabriel Cousens' Tree of Life Rejuvenation Center. He showed the audience how to make raw "pizza" and talked about the benefits of a raw food diet. When he passed around samples, she was hooked on the taste, but more so on the significance of the event—it was *healthy* food!

She learned all she could about food and nutrition, taking numerous workshops and training with others who were enthused about a healthy food lifestyle. She spent two years at the world-famous Living Light Culinary Institute, the world's premier raw food culinary school, as Executive Assistant to the Director, Cherie Soria, and she devoted three years to training to become a Certified Nutritionist.

Over the decades, Chef Colleen has partnered with many other chefs, nutritionists, and healers to integrate optimal nutrition and wellness into peoples' diets and health regimens. As the "Resident Superfood Chef" for David Wolfe's Longevity Now® Conferences, and with Jing Herbs, she created and published hundreds of superfood and herbal recipes to support health, beauty, and longevity. She has worked with many top names in the health industry, winning awards for her recipes. She has also helped organize numerous conferences around healthy nutrition. Chef Colleen has launched "Tonic Bars" in cities around the world, serving thousands of customers.

Currently, she teaches classes, coaches individuals, and consults with clients ranging from restaurants, cafes, and food trucks to juice bars, mail order companies and acupuncture clinics.

ACKNOWLEDGMENTS

Dr. John

I thank my publishers, Rick Benzel and Susan Shankin, for making such a book happen. They connected me with Chef Colleen Cackowski whose delicious recipes are the backbone of this book. Thank you so much Colleen for your creative and unique recipes that show people how they can easily make grain-free meals that keep their blood sugar low.

I thank Rick and Susan for their excellent work in editing and designing the book. Thanks also to the following people who contributed to the book in many ways:

- Elizabeth Lenthall for her assistance in helping with this cookbook including editing the recipes, being an art director at the photo shoot, and designing interior pages.
- Julie Simpson for her copyediting of the manuscript.
- Diya Loney for her tasty warm salad dressing recipes.
- Anthony Nex for the beautiful photos of Chef Colleen's recipes. Food stylist Diane Elander and prop stylist Kristine Nex for their creative work during the photo shoot.
- Darcy Hughes and Felipe Zamora for their promotional marketing work.

Finally, I thank my wife of 50 years, Maria Poothullil, for her patience and support as I endeavor to challenge the theory of insulin resistance and propose a new way to explain the real cause of Type 2 diabetes and the right cure through my books and speaking engagements.

Chef Colleen

I thank my mother, Eileen, for inspiring and teaching me, as a seven-year-old, how to cook. Now, making good food has become a passion that serves not only me, but those around me.

I also thank my mentor, Abdy, and my friend Tracey, whose love, support and guidance made it possible for me to contribute to this book.

And I thank Dr. John for standing up and sharing your unique viewpoint and inspiring people to bring about a healthier world in a delicious way!

OTHER BOOKS ON DIABETES BY DR. JOHN POOTHULLIL

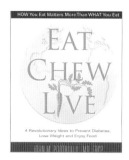

Eat Chew Live: 4 Revolutionary Ideas to Prevent Diabetes, Lose Weight and Enjoy Food. This book goes into extensive detail about the lack of logic with the insulin resistance theory as the cause of high blood sugar and Type 2 diabetes, and what everyone can do to change their thinking and eating habits.

Winner, 2016 Beverly Hills Books Awards

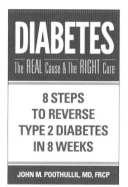

Diabetes—The Real Cause and The Right Cure: 8 Steps to Reverse Type 2 Diabetes in 8 Weeks. This book explains the background science about how the overconsumption of grains is the real cause of Type 2 diabetes and provides 8 clear steps you can take to reverse an existing condition, including diet and exercise.

Finalist, 2017 Beverly Hills Books Awards, Diet & Nutrition Category

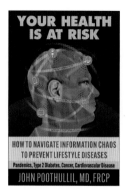

Your Health Is at Risk: How to Navigate Information Chaos to Prevent Lifestyle. This book explains how medical disinformation, misinformation, and missing Information (DMMI) are increasingly pervasive in the media and social media, leading you to make poor or wrong decisions about your lifestyle choices and healthcare. The book offers insights into how you can making wiser decisions based on science to improve your health.

Gold Medal Winner, 2023 Nautilus Book Awards and Independent Press (Ippy) Awards.